PRINCIPAL DRUGS

Principal Drugs

An Alphabetical Guide

S. J. HOPKINS F.P.S.

Consultant Pharmacist,
Addenbrooke's Hospital, Cambridge

with a foreword by

C. A. KEELE M.D., F.R.C.P.

Professor of Pharmacology and
Therapeutics, University of London

FABER AND FABER
3 Queen Square
London

First published in 1958
by Faber and Faber Limited
3 Queen Square London WC1
Second edition 1964
Third edition 1969
Reprinted 1970
Fourth edition 1973
Reprinted 1975, 1976
Fifth edition 1977
Printed in Great Britain by
Butler & Tanner Ltd, Frome and London

ISBN 0 571 04938 9

Preface to First Edition

The aim of this small dictionary is to provide nurses and others with a brief account of some of the more important drugs in common use. The larger works on drugs and their actions are well known but expensive, and are not always readily accessible to nurses. The smaller books on pharmacology do not deal with the subject in the same way, so it is hoped that this book will bridge the gap, and serve as a concise guide to drugs in current use.

Many drugs are prescribed under proprietary names, and such names are indicated by an initial capital letter. Where an approved non-proprietary name exists, the drug is described under that name, and a cross-reference is given from the proprietary name by the abbreviation, *q.v.* (which see). The physical limitations of a book of this size do not permit the inclusion of all the proprietary names that may exist for any one drug, but omissions are entirely arbitrary, and do not reflect in any way upon the products concerned.

In contrast to many other reference books, doses are given either in the imperial or metric systems, but not in both. The doses of the older drugs such as digitalis are expressed in the imperial system, as it is in that system that these drugs are usually prescribed. Conversely, the doses of the newer drugs are given in the metric system. There seems little point in giving imperial doses of those drugs which are prescribed and dispensed solely in metric terms. Comments on this or any other aspect of the book will be welcomed.   S. J. H.

1958

Preface to Fifth Edition

The aim of this small dictionary of drugs is to provide nurses and others interested in medicinal products with a concise guide to some of the drugs in current use. Proprietary names of drugs are indicated by a capital initial letter, but the drug concerned is described under its 'approved' or non-proprietary name, which has a small initial letter. A cross-reference from the proprietary name to the approved name is given by the abbreviation, *q.v.*

In a book of this limited size, it is impossible to describe all the drugs in current use, and only rarely is reference made to any mixed product. For the same reason, proprietary names are not given in the description of the drug, as several brands of the same drug may be available. In the great majority of cases, if either the 'approved' or proprietary name of the drug is known, the alternative name can be found by reference to the List of Approved and Proprietary Names on page 113. In this edition, the value of this List has been increased by including in both parts of the List a very brief indication of the main use of the drug, so even if a drug is not described in the main part of the book, its name and use may well be mentioned in this extended List of Names.

Doses also present some problems, as different doses may be given on occasion for different purposes. In general, only standard adult doses are referred to, usually given three or four times a day, but as a rule, if a dose is referred to as 'daily', it should be understood as being given in smaller divided doses during the day, and not as a single daily dose.

S. J. H.

1976

Foreword

The number of drugs used in medicine today continues to increase as new and important discoveries are made. It is becoming increasingly difficult even for doctors to learn and remember the names and uses of all the available drugs. For nurses it must be a well-nigh impossible task. I am therefore very happy to welcome this book by Mr S. J. Hopkins, who has provided just the sort of information which nurses are likely to want. Both old and new drugs are listed in alphabetical order and concise notes on actions, uses and doses are given in each case. I forecast that this book will fulfil a great need.

C. A. KEELE

1958

Contents

Weights and Measures

Metric System

microgram (mcg) or 0·001 mg
milligram (mg) or 0·001 g
centigram (cg) or 0·01 g
decigram (dg) or 0·1 g
gram (g). (In prescriptions the abbreviation
       'G' was formerly preferred.)
kilogram (kg) = 1,000 grams

The only metric measures of capacity which the nurse is
likely to meet are the
     millilitre (ml) which is approximately equal to
       the cubic centimetre (cc)
litre (1) = 1,000 ml or cc

Imperial System

(No longer used for prescriptions)

grain
ounce   = 437·5 grains
pound (lb) = 16 oz = 7,000 grains

minim
ounce   = 480 minims
pint   = 20 fluid oz

Approximate Imperial and Metric equivalents

1 grain	= 60 mg
1 ounce (oz)	= 28·4 g
1 pound	= 453 g
1 fl. oz	= 28·4 ml or cc
1 pint	= 568 ml or cc
1 mg	= $\frac{1}{60}$ grain
100 mg	= $1\frac{1}{2}$ grains
1 gram	= 15 grains
1 kg	= 2·2 pounds
1 ml	= 16·9 minims
100 ml	= 3·5 ounces
1 litre	= 35 ounces

Abbreviations Used in Prescriptions

The use of Latin abbreviations in prescription-writing is no longer recommended, and both the name of the drug, and the directions for use, should be written in English, and in full. The use of some time-hallowed abbreviations still persists, and the following list is a selection of those terms that may be met with.

---

aa.	ana	of each
a.c.	ante cibum	before food
aq.	aqua	water
arg.	argentum	silver
b.d.	bis die	twice a day
c.	cum	with
collut.	collutorium	mouthwash
collyr.	collyrium	eye lotion
crem.	cremor	cream
et	et	and
ft.	fiat	make
fer.	ferrum	iron
garg.	gargarisma	gargle
gtt.	guttae	drops
liq.	liquor	solution
lot.	lotio	lotion
mist.	mistura	mixture
mitt.	mitte	send
moll.	molle	soft
narist.	naristillae	nasal drops
neb.	nebula	spray
oculent.	oculentum	eye ointment
o.n.	omni nocte	every night

p.a.a.	*parti affectae applicandus*	apply to the affected part
p.aeq.	*partes aequales*	equal parts
p.c.	*post cibum*	after food
p.r.n.	*pro re nata*	occasionally
pig.	*pigmentum*	paint
q.d.	*quater die*	four times a day
q.q.h.	*quarta quaque hora*	every four hours
q.s.	*quantum sufficiat*	sufficient
s.o.s.	*si opus sit*	when necessary
stat.	*statim*	at once
supp.	*suppositorium*	suppository
t.d.s.	*ter die sumendus*	to be taken three times a day
t.i.d.	*ter in die*	three times a day
ung.	*unguentum*	ointment

DICTIONARY OF DRUGS

A

A.C.T.H. Corticotrophin, *q.v.*

A.P.T. Alum precipitated diphtheria toxoid. A diphtheria prophylactic for young children. Initial dose 0·5 ml, by intramuscular or deep subcutaneous injection, followed by 0·5 ml, not less than four weeks later.

A.T.10. A solution of dihydrotachysterol. It increases blood-calcium by mobilizing calcium from bone, and is used in tetany due to parathyroid deficiency and in rickets not responding to calciferol. Initial dose 3 ml, maintenance dose 0·5 to 1 ml daily together with calcium gluconate or lactate.

acebutolol. A beta-blocking agent with a more cardio-selective action than propranolol and some associated drugs, and is less likely to cause bronchospasm. Chiefly indicated in angina and cardiac arrhythmias. Dose 200 mg twice daily, but larger doses may be required. Can be given intravenously in doses of 25 mg in severe arrhythmias.

acetarsol. An organic arsenic compound used in the treatment of amoebiasis in doses of 250 mg twice or thrice daily for 7 to 10 days, usually with emetine. Pessaries containing 250 mg are used in trichomonal vaginitis. It may cause cutaneous reactions.

acetazolamide. A mild diuretic, now used mainly in glaucoma. It decreases intraocular pressure by reducing the formation of aqueous humour. Dose, 250 mg four times a day.

acetohexamide. An orally active hypoglycaemic drug similar in action to tolbutamide, *q.v.* Mainly indicated in the middle-aged late-onset type of diabetic. Dose, 250 mg to 1 g daily as a single morning dose. Side-effects include gastro-intestinal disturbances, skin rashes and headache.

acetomenaphthone. An orally active synthetic vitamin K. It is used in haemorrhage due to prothrombin deficiency, and in the pre-operative treatment of obstructive jaundice, in doses of 10 to 20 mg daily. Also of value in prophylaxis against neonatal haemorrhage when given in doses of 1 to 10 mg daily before delivery.

acetophenetidin. Phenacetin, *q.v.*

acetylsalicylic acid. Aspirin, *q.v.*

Achromycin. Tetracycline, *q.v.*

acriflavine. Orange-red dye with antiseptic properties. Used as lotion 1:1,000. Acriflavine emulsion is a bland application containing liquid paraffin. Proflavine and euflavine are related compounds.

actinomycin D. An antibiotic with cytostatic properties used in Hodgkin's disease, in Wilm's tumour and other malignant tumours. Dose 0.5 mg intravenously daily for five days. It also has immunosuppressive properties and is used with other drugs in transplant surgery to reduce the risks of rejection. It has a toxic effect on the bone marrow, and care is necessary in assessing dose and duration of treatment.

adrenaline. Known in the U.S. as epinephrine, adrenaline is one of the blood-pressure-raising principles of the adrenal gland. Now prepared synthetically. The pressor effect is due to a constriction of the peripheral blood-vessels, and an increase in cardiac output. It may cause ventricular fibrillation if given during halothane, cyclopropane, or trichlorethylene anaesthesia. In hypotensive crises, noradrenaline, *q.v.*, or metaraminol, *q.v.*, are preferred, as the intravenous use of adrenaline is potentially dangerous. It is added to local anaesthetic solutions (1:50,000 to 1:200,000) to reduce diffusion and prolong the anaesthetic effect. It also has a powerful bronchodilator action, and is given as a 1:1,000 solution by subcutaneous injection (0·2 to 0·5 ml) to relieve asthmatic attacks, serum sickness, urticaria, etc., occasionally applied locally to stop capillary bleeding and epistaxis. It has been used by intracardiac injection (0·25 ml) in cardiac arrest and syncope.

Solutions of adrenaline may darken on storage and lose activity.

Adriamycin. Doxorubicin, *q.v.*

Aerosporin. Polymyxin, *q.v.*

agar. The gelatinous extract obtained from certain seaweeds. Used as a bulk laxative. Dose 4 to 16 g.

Akineton. Biperiden, *q.v.*

Albamycin. Novobiocin, *q.v.*

Albucid. Sulphacetamide, *q.v.*

alcohol (ethanol). It is used occasionally by injection to destroy nerve tissue in the treatment of intractable trigeminal neuralgia. Industrial alcohol or methylated spirit contains 5% of wood naphtha; surgical spirit is industrial spirit with the addition of castor oil, methyl salicylate and other substances and is used for skin preparation and the prevention of pressure sores. Commercial methylated spirit contains pyridine, and is coloured with methyl violet, and is not suitable for medical purposes.

Alcopar. Bephenium, *q.v.*

alcuronium. A muscle-relaxant similar to tubocurarine. It causes less histamine release and consequent fall in blood-pressure. Dose 10 to 15 mg intravenously, repeated as required with doses of 3 to 5 mg. Reduced doses should be given during halothane, ether or cyclopropane anaesthesia.

Aldactone. Spironolactone, q.v.

Aldomet. Methyldopa, q.v.

aldosterone. The main mineralo-corticoid hormone of the adrenal cortex. Given by intravenous injection in doses of 0·5 mg in severe Addison's disease. An excessive secretion of aldosterone may occur in some oedematous states and inhibit the action of thiazide diuretics, and spironolactone, q.v., can suppress such inhibition, and increase diuresis.

Alevaire. A solution of tyloxapol used by inhalation to reduce excessive or thickened bron-cho-pulmonary secretions in asthma, bronchiectasis, and post-operative pulmonary conditions.

Alkeran. Melphalan, q.v.

Allegron. Nortriptyline, q.v.

Alloferin. Alcuronium, q.v.

allopurinol. An enzyme inhibitor that blocks the formation of uric acid, and so is useful in the treatment of chronic gout. Dose 200 to 600 mg daily after initial doses of 50 mg. Also useful in the hyperuricaemia of leukaemia. Side-effects in-clude nausea, headache and pruritus.

aloes. A powerful cathartic, and is usually given with carminatives to prevent grip-ing. Dose 100 to 300 mg.

Althesin. A steroid preparation characterized by its unusual anaesthetic properties. Used for induction, or as the main anaesthetic for short opera-tions. Dose 0·05 to 0·075 ml per kg body-weight by slow intravenous injection.

Aludrox. A preparation of alu-minium hydroxide, q.v.

alum. Used for its astringent properties as a mouth-wash (1 to 2%); as a douche (0·5%); and as a lotion (2%).

aluminium. The powdered metal is used as a skin protective in ileostomy, as Baltimore paste, q.v., also known as Com-pound Aluminium Paste.

aluminium hydroxide. An antacid with a prolonged action. Unlike the carbonates, it does not liberate carbon dioxide, is not absorbed and so does not cause alkalosis. Given in suspension as a gel (dose 7·5 to 15 ml), or as tab-lets of the dried gel (500 mg). Dose 1 to 2 tablets, chewed or crushed before swallowing.

Alupent. Orciprenaline, q.v.

amantadine. An antiviral drug, used in prophylaxis against some forms of influenza. It is also used in parkinsonism, and in association with other drugs, may give valuable symptomatic relief. Dose 200 mg daily.

Ambilhar. Niridazole, *q.v.*

amethocaine hydrochloride. Local anaesthetic, used for anaesthesia of mucous membranes 1 to 2% solution; eyedrops 0·25 to 1%. As spray for throat before endoscopy etc., 0·5% solution may be used. The toxic effects are similar to those of cocaine.

amiloride. A diuretic with an action on the distal tubule similar to that of spironolactone, *q.v.*, increasing sodium excretion, but reducing potassium loss. Dose 10 to 40 mg daily.

aminocaproic acid. An antifibrinolytic drug, used in the treatment of haemorrhage due to an excessive breakdown of fibrin, and in haematuria following prostatectomy. Dose 4 to 6 g initially, followed by 1 g hourly, orally or by slow intravenous injection.

aminophylline. Theophylline with ethylenediamine. It is more soluble and less irritant than theophylline, but may cause gastric disturbance. It relaxes involuntary muscle and stimulates respiration and heart rate. It is used mainly in congestive heart failure, asthma and cardiac and renal oedema. Useful by injection

in Cheyne-Stokes breathing. Tablets of 0·1 g; ampoules (intramuscular) 0·5 g in 2 ml; ampoules (intravenous) 0·25 g in 10 ml and suppositories of 0·36 g.

aminosalicylic acid. Para-aminosalicylic acid, *q.v.*

Aminosol. A solution containing a mixture of amino-acids and peptides, obtained by the hydrolysis of protein. It is specially prepared for intravenous use to supply the equivalent of protein when food cannot be taken by mouth. Also available with dextrose and alcohol when additional calories are required. Several preparations of pure amino-acids, represented by Trophysan, are also available.

amitriptyline. A tricyclic antidepressant drug similar in action to imipramine *q.v.*, but apart from causing dryness of the mouth and drowsiness, it has few side-effects. Dose 25 mg thrice daily. Maximum benefit may not be obtained until after 3–6 weeks' treatment, and prolonged use may be necessary to prevent relapse. Contra-indicated in glaucoma, prostatic hypertrophy and pregnancy.

ammonium chloride. A mild expectorant and diuretic, sometimes given in association with mandelic acid in urinary infections. Dose 300 mg to 2 g.

amodiaquine. An anti-malarial of high potency and low toxicity. A weekly dose of 400 mg is given for suppressive treatment; for relief of an attack a dose of 600 mg followed by a dose of 400 mg daily for two days may be given. Has caused corneal deposits and pigmentation of the nails and skin when given for long periods.

Amoxil. Amoxycillin, q.v.

amoxycillin. A wide-range orally-active penicillin derivative used in the treatment of respiratory, urinary and soft tissue infections. Dose 250 to 500 mg.

amphetamine sulphate. A powerful central nervous system stimulant. Has been used in depressive states and narcolepsy, but dependence may occur and it is now rarely prescribed.

amphotericin B. An antifungal antibiotic, effective in systemic as well as superficial infections. For systemic use it is given by slow intravenous drip infusion in a dose of 0·1 mg per kg body-weight; locally as lotion, cream or pessaries.

ampicillin. An orally active penicillin derivative with a range of activity similar to tetracycline, as it is effective against many Gram-negative as well as Gram-positive organisms. It is widely used in chronic bronchitis and infections of the biliary and urinary tracts, but may cause skin reactions. Dose 250 to 500 mg, six-hourly. Of no value against penicillinase-producing organisms.

amylobarbitone. A barbiturate of medium intensity. Dose 100 to 200 mg. Sodium derivative is more rapid in action, but the effect less prolonged; occasionally given by intravenous injection.

Amytal. Amylobarbitone, q.v.

Anahaemin. A highly refined extract of liver used mainly in the treatment of macrocytic anaemias that do not respond to cyanocobalamin alone. Dose 2 to 4 ml by intramuscular injection.

Anapolon. Oxymetholone, q.v.

ancrod. An anticoagulant obtained from the venom of a Malayan viper. It alters fibrinogen so that it does not react with thrombin to form fibrin, and any fibrin formed by other factors in the blood is rapidly removed by plasmin. The lower fibrinogen levels reduce blood viscosity, and the long action of ancrod allows a smooth change to oral anticoagulants. Of value in deep vein thrombosis, embolism and vascular surgery. Dose 2 to 3 units/kg by intravenous infusion, repeated as needed.

Anectine. Suxamethonium, *q.v.*

Anethaine. Amethocaine, *q.v.*

aneurine hydrochloride. Thiamine, *q.v.*

Anquil. Benperidol, *q.v.*

Ansolysen. Pentolinium, *q.v.*

Antabuse. Disulfiram, *q.v.*

antazoline. Antihistamine drug similar to but less active than mepyramine, *q.v.* Dose 100 to 200 mg.

Antepar. A preparation of piperazine, *q.v.*

Anthipen. Dichlorophen, *q.v.*

Anthisan. Mepyramine maleate, *q.v.*

antibiotics. Antibacterial substances which occur as by-products of the growth of certain moulds. The first to be discovered was penicillin, derived from *Penicillium notatum*. It remains the drug of choice in the treatment of many infections due to Gram-positive organisms. Penicillin is remarkable also for its low toxicity. Streptomycin was next introduced but is much more toxic than penicillin and it is used chiefly in tuberculosis. Further research has resulted in the discovery of aureomycin, chloramphenicol, erythromycin, the tetracyclines and the cephaloridine group of antibiotics. Some penicillin derivatives (ampicillin, *q.v.*) have a wide range of activity; others (cloxacillin, *q.v.* and flucloxacillin, *q.v.*) are markedly effective against resistant staphylococci, and carbenicillin, *q.v.* is effective against *Pseudomonas pyocyanea*. Gentamicin, q.v., and colistin, *q.v.*, represent antibiotics of value in infections due to Gram-negative organisms, and rifampicin is effective in tuberculosis. Wide-range antibiotics should not be given for more than 5–10 days, as otherwise the normal bacterial flora of the intestines may be disturbed, leading to overgrowth of fungal organisms such as monilia.

Certain antibiotics, including neomycin and bacitracin, are too toxic for systemic use, but may be useful in the treatment of infected skin conditions.

The systemic antibiotics, if used for external application, should be used for short periods only, as they may give rise to skin irritation and sensitization. A few antibiotics such as doxorubicin, *q.v.*, have cytostatic properties.

antimony and potassium tartrate. Used in the tropical helminth diseases schistosomiasis and leishmaniasis. Dose 30 mg by intravenous injection initially, increased slowly by increments of 30 mg to 120 mg, and to a total dose of 1·5 g.

Antistin. Antazoline, *q.v.*

antitoxic sera. The serum of animals containing antibodies or antitoxins. When such serum is injected, it confers a temporary immunity against certain bacterial toxins. The principal antitoxic sera include diphtheria antitoxin and tetanus antitoxin. The use of sera has markedly declined with the introduction of sulphonamides and antibiotics.

Antrypol. Suramin, *q.v.*

Anturan. Sulphinpyrazone, *q.v.*

apomorphine. A morphine derivative with a rapid and powerful emetic action when injected. Dose 2 to 8 mg by subcutaneous injection.

Apresoline. Hydrallazine, *q.v.*

Aprinox. Bendrofluazide, *q.v.*

Aprotinon. An inactivator of pancreatic enzymes, used in pancreatitis and fibrinolytic haemorrhage. Dose 50,000 to 100,000 units intravenously.

Aquamephyton. Vitamin K, *q.v.*

arachis oil. Ground-nut or peanut oil. It resembles olive oil in its emollient properties, and is used in dermatology to soften the crusts of eczema and psoriasis, often in conjunction with calamine.

Aramine. Metaraminol, *q.v.*

Arfonad. Trimetaphan, *q.v.*

Arlef. Flufenamic acid, *q.v.*

Artane. Benzhexol hydrochloride, *q.v.*

Arvin. Ancrod, *q.v.*

ascorbic acid (vitamin C). Present in many citrus fruits. Used in some anaemias, but deficiency is unusual with normal diet. Severe deficiency causes scurvy. Prophylactic dose 25 to 75 mg daily; therapeutic dose 200 to 500 mg daily.

aspirin. Acetylsalicylic acid. Widely used as a mild analgesic and anti-inflammatory agent, often in association with other drugs such as paracetamol and codeine. Dose 300 mg to 1 g, but in acute and chronic rheumatoid conditions doses of 4 to 8 g daily have been given for long periods. Side-effects include gastric irritation with some blood loss, tinnitus and hyperventilation. The blood loss may cause anaemia if treatment is prolonged. Aspirin may also cause bronchospasm in asthmatic and other sensitive patients. Excessive and prolonged use, especially when given with phenacetin, *q.v.*, may cause 'analgesic nephropathy'. Soluble aspirin tablets contain chalk to reduce the local irritant effects, and although a paediatric aspirin tablet is available, aspirin should not be given to children under one year of age. Aspirin may increase the effects of certain hypoglycaemic and anticoagulant drugs. The anti-inflammatory action has been ascribed to the inhibition of prostaglandin (*q.v.*) synthesis.

Atromid-S. Clofibrate, *q.v.*

Ativan. Lorazepam, *q.v.*

atropine. An alkaloid obtained from belladonna, hyoscyamus and other plants. Powerful antispasmodic, mydriatic, and central nervous system depressant. Often given by injection with morphine for pre-operative sedation. Contra-indicated in glaucoma. Dose 0·25 to 2 mg.

atropine methonitrate. A less toxic derivative of atropine; used orally as an antispasmodic in asthma, bronchospasm, pylorospasm and similar conditions. Dose 1 to 2 mg.

aureomycin. Chlortetracycline, *q.v.*

Aventyl. Nortriptyline, *q.v.*

Avloclor. Chloroquine, *q.v.*

Avomine. Derivative of promethazine, *q.v.*, used in travel sickness, vomiting of pregnancy, etc. Dose 25 mg.

azathioprine. A compound with cytostatic properties, as it is slowly converted to mercaptopurine, *q.v.*, in the body. Of value as an immunosuppressive agent in preventing the rejection of renal and other transplanted organs, in association with large doses of prednisone. Dose 2 to 5 mg per kg body-weight daily.

B

B.A.L. Dimercaprol, *q.v.*

B.I.P.P. A mixture of bismuth subnitrate, iodoform, and liquid paraffin. Occasionally used as an antiseptic dressing, applied on gauze.

bacitracin. An antibiotic used by local application in skin diseases due to Gram-positive organisms resistant to other forms of treatment. It is too toxic for systemic use.

baclofen. A relaxant of voluntary muscle, useful in multiple sclerosis and the muscle spasm of spinal lesions. Dose 5 mg initially, maintenance doses 40 to 60 mg daily.

Bactrim. Referred to under trimethoprim, *q.v.*

baltimore paste. Compound Aluminium Paste B.P.C. Contains aluminium powder, zinc oxide and liquid paraffin. It is used as a skin protective in ileostomy and gastric fistula.

Banocide. Diethylcarbamazine, *q.v.*

barbitone. One of the earliest of the group of hypnotic drugs known generically as the barbiturates. The use of barbiturates is declining as safer drugs are now available. Dose 300 to 600 mg.

barium sulphate. A very insoluble powder, given orally or rectally as an aqueous suspension as contrast agent for X-ray examination of the alimentary system. *Note:— Soluble* salts of barium are very poisonous.

Baycaron. Mefruside, *q.v.*

beclamide. An anticonvulsant used in grand mal and psychomotor epilepsy. May be given in association with phenobarbitone. Dose 0·5 to 1 g.

beclomethasone. A synthetic corticosteroid for topical application in inflamed skin conditions. Used as ointment or cream (0·025%), often with neomycin. Also used by inhalation in asthma.

Becotide. A preparation of beclomethasone, *q.v.*, for inhalation in the treatment of asthma. May permit the reduction or withdrawal of systemic steroids.

Beflavit. Riboflavine, *q.v.*

belladonna. The dried leaves of deadly nightshade (*Atropa belladonna*). The principal constituent is atropine, *q.v.* Used in colic, peptic ulcer, whooping cough and enuresis. Dose of tincture of belladonna 0·5 to 2 ml.

bemegride. A barbiturate antagonist, occasionally used in the treatment of barbiturate poisoning. Dose of 50 mg by intravenous injection, repeated up to a total dose of 1 g.

Benadon. Pyridoxine, *q.v.*

Benadryl. Diphenhydramine, *q.v.*

benapryzine. A spasmolytic agent used in parkinsonism and similar drug-induced conditions. May be given with levodopa or amantadine if necessary. Dose 150 to 200 mg daily.

bendrofluazide. A diuretic of the chlorothiazide type, but with a more powerful and prolonged action. Used in congestive heart failure, oedema, and in hypertension to potentiate the action of other drugs. Give potassium supplements with prolonged treatment. Dose 2·5 to 10 mg daily.

Benemid. Probenecid, *q.v.*

Benerva. Thiamine hydrochloride, *q.v.*

Benoral. Benorylate, *q.v.*

benorylate. A derivative of aspirin and paracetamol, with the general properties of both drugs. Used in arthritic conditions and for the relief of painful musculoskeletal disorders. Like aspirin, it may cause gastro-intestinal disturbance and other side-effects. It may increase the action of oral anticoagulants.

benperidol. A tranquillizer for use in controlling antisocial sexual behaviour. Dose 0·25 to 1·5 mg daily.

benzalkonium chloride. A detergent with antiseptic properties, used mainly for skin preparation, and for the storage of instruments.

benzhexol hydrochloride. A spasmolytic drug with atropine-like properties used mainly to relieve the tremor and rigidity of parkinsonism. Initial doses should be small, increased gradually until the optimum effect is obtained. Side-effects include dryness of the mouth, and with high doses, psychotic disturbances may occur. Dose 2 to 20 mg daily.

benzocaine. A local anaesthetic for topical application. Used as lozenges (100 mg) for painful oral conditions; ointment (5 to 10%); suppositories 200 mg.

benzoctamine. A tranquillizing agent used in anxiety and tension states. Dose 10 mg.

benzoic acid. It has fungistatic properties similar to salicylic acid, and is used as Whitfield's ointment (Compound Benzoic Acid Ointment) for the treatment of ringworm.

benzoin. A balsamic resin. Widely used in the treatment of bronchitis, pharyngitis and catarrh by steam inhalation of friar's balsam (Compound Tincture of Benzoin).

benztropine. A spasmolytic drug used to relieve the rigidity, muscle spasm, tremor and salivation of Parkinson's disease. Less likely to cause mental disturbance than benzhexol, *q.v.* Dose 0·5 to 6 mg daily.

benzyl benzoate. A clear liquid with an aromatic odour. It is used as an emulsion in the treatment of scabies; two applications to the whole of the body except the head being sufficient to eliminate the parasites.

benzyl penicillin. Penicillin, *q.v.*

bephenium. An anthelmintic effective against hookworm and roundworm. Given as a single dose of 5 g on an empty stomach. A second dose may be given later if necessary.

beta-adrenergic blocking agents. Adrenaline and related catecholamines are released into the circulation during exercise and stress, and stimulate cardiac output by acting on the beta-adrenoreceptor sites in the heart. When such stimulation is excessive, it may cause myocardial insufficiency and angina. Drugs such as propranolol, *q.v.*, block these receptor sites and so indirectly reduce cardiac stimulation, and are of value in the control of angina. Some also act on other receptor sites and may cause broncho-spasm by releasing histamine. Newer drugs, represented by acebutolol, *q.v.*, and meto-prolol, are more cardio-selective, and others such as sotalol, *q.v.*, are of more value in hypertension. By the nature of these drugs, care is necessary in heart block and cardio-genic shock.

Beta-Cardone. Sotalol, *q.v.*

Betadine. A complex of iodine with povidone. The combination slowly breaks down in contact with the skin and mucous surfaces to liberate free iodine, which has power-ful antiseptic properties. The complex is useful for pre-operative skin preparation, and infected wounds.

betahistine. A vasodilator with some of the properties of histamine. Used to reduce the vertigo of Ménière's disease. Should be used with care in asthmatics. Dose 8 to 48 mg daily.

Betaloc. Metoprolol, *q.v.*

betamethasone. A synthetic corticosteroid of the cortisone type, but is characterized by the low dose, increased anti-inflammatory action, and reduced side-effects. It has virtually no salt-retaining properties, and causes little increase in the urinary excre-tion of potassium. Indicated

in all conditions requiring corticosteroid therapy, with the exception of Addison's disease and after adrenalec-tomy when a salt-retaining steroid is required. Dose 0·5 to 5 mg daily in divided doses. Preparations for topical use are also available.

bethanidine. A hypotensive drug that functions by a selective blocking of impulses in the sympathetic nervous system. Useful in severe hypertension, or when guanethidine or re-lated drugs are not well toler-ated. Dose 20 to 200 mg daily.

Betnelan. Betamethasone, *q.v.*

Betnovate. Betamethasone, *q.v.*

Biligrafin. A radio-opaque diagnostic agent. Given by intravenous injection for X-ray visualization of the biliary tract.

Biogastrone. Carbenoxolone, *q.v.*

biperiden. An antispasmodic and parasympatholytic drug, used chiefly to control the rigidity and excessive saliva-tion of parkinsonism. It has less effect on tremor. Dose 1 to 2 mg, increased as required up to 12 mg daily.

bisacodyl. A synthetic laxative that exerts its action by a direct stimulating effect on the nerve endings of the colon. Dose 10 mg orally, or as a suppository.

bismuth subgallate. A yellow

insoluble powder with astringent properties. Used as dusting powder, and as suppositories for rectal conditions.

bismuth subnitrate. A constituent of B.I.P.P. (bismuth, iodoform and paraffin paste), occasionally used as an antiseptic application.

Bisolvon. Bromhexine, *q.v.*

bleomycin. An antibiotic with cytotoxic properties. Exceptional in causing little if any disturbance of bone marrow activity. Used mainly in skin tumours, lymphomas, and mycosis fungoides. Dose 15 to 30 mg twice weekly by intramuscular or intravenous injection.

Blocadren. Timolol, *q.v.*

Bolvidon. Mianserin, *q.v.*

boric acid, boracic acid. Mild antiseptic. Should not be applied to large, raw areas owing to risk of absorption in toxic amounts.

Bradosol. Domiphen, *q.v.*

Breoprin. Aspirin, *q.v.*

Brevidil. Suxamethonium, *q.v.*

Bricanyl. Terbutaline, *q.v.*

Brietal. Methohexitone, *q.v.*

brilliant green. An antiseptic dye occasionally used as a lotion, 1 in 1,000; also as an ointment (2%).

Brinaldix. Clopamide, *q.v.*

Brizin. Benapryzine, *q.v.*

bromhexine. An expectorant with mucolytic properties. It reduces the viscosity of purulent sputum, and stimulates the production of thin, easily expectorated sputum. Useful in acute and chronic bronchitis when tenacious sputum complicates treatment. Dose 8 mg.

bromocriptine. A new type of therapeutic agent with a marked effect on the action of the pituitary gland. It is used at present for the inhibition of lactation, but may have wider applications in unrelated conditions associated with pituitary dysfunction. Dose, 2·5 mg twice daily with food for 14 days.

Broxil. Phenethicillin, *q.v.*

Brufen. Ibuprofen, *q.v.*

bumetanide. A diuretic similar to frusemide, *q.v.* Dose 1 to 4 mg daily.

bupivacaine. A local anaesthetic related to lignocaine, but characterized by its increased potency and long duration of action. Used as a 0·25 to 0·5 per cent solution, with adrenaline, for nerve block analgesia.

Burinex. Bumetanide, *q.v.*

Buscopan. Hyoscine butylbromide, *q.v.*

busulphan. A cytostatic compound with a selective action on the bone marrow, and used in the palliative treatment of chronic myeloid leukaemia. Close haematological control is essential during treatment as remission of symptoms may not be complete for some weeks. Dose 0·5 to 4 mg daily.

Butazolidin. Phenylbutazone, *q.v.*

butobarbitone. A barbiturate of medium intensity and rapidity of onset. Dose 60 to 200 mg.

C

C.T.A.B. Cetrimide, *q.v.*

caffeine. The central nervous system stimulant present in tea and coffee. It is used with paracetamol and other mild analgesics for headache. Caffeine also has some mild diuretic action. Dose 250 to 500 mg. Caffeine sodium benzoate is a soluble compound used by injection as a cardiac and respiratory stimulant. Dose 0·3 to 1 g.

calamine. Zinc carbonate. It has a mild astringent and soothing action when applied to the skin, and is widely used as Calamine Lotion for skin irritation and as Oily Calamine Lotion in eczema.

calciferol (vitamin D_2). Vitamin D is essential for the absorption of calcium and phosphorus from the diet. Deficiency in infants may lead to rickets and poor tooth development. Prophylactic dose 800 units daily, therapeutic doses 5,000 to 50,000 units. Larger doses are used in para-

thyroid deficiency, but prolonged high-dose treatment may cause hypercalcaemia, calcium deposition in the kidneys and other toxic effects.

Calcitare. Calcitonin, *q.v.*

calcitonin. A hormone of the thyroid gland, which has an action similar to that of the parathyroid gland in regulating blood calcium levels. Given in the hypercalcaemia due to tumours, in osteoporosis, and in Paget's disease. Dose may vary from 10 to 160 units daily by injection.

calcium alginate. A substance derived from seaweed that can be made into fibres resembling cotton wool or gauze. It has haemostatic properties, and may be applied to bleeding surfaces, or used to pack cavities. It is slowly absorbed by the tissues if left in position.

calcium chloride. Has the general action of calcium salts, but it is irritating orally; intramuscular injections cause local necrosis, and intravenous injections must be given very slowly to avoid reactions. Calcium gluconate, *q.v.*, is sometimes preferred.

calcium gluconate. A calcium salt used in many conditions associated with calcium deficiency such as tetany, rickets, coeliac disease, parathyroid deficiency, and during pregnancy and lactation often in association with vitamin D. Calcium gluconate is also given in chilblains, urticaria and allergic reactions. The drug may be given orally, intramuscularly as a 10% solution, or in emergency by slow intravenous injection. Dose 1 to 5 g.

calcium lactate. Given in calcium-deficiency states, but calcium gluconate is usually preferred. Dose 1 to 5 g.

Camcolit. Lithium carbonate, *q.v.*

capreomycin. An antibiotic of value in resistant tuberculosis or when other antibiotics are not tolerated. May cause tinnitus and renal damage. Dose 1 g daily by intramuscular injection.

carbachol. A parasympathomimetic agent used orally and by injection in the treatment of post-operative atony and retention of urine, and occasionally as eye-drops in the treatment of glaucoma. Dose 2 to 4 mg orally, 0·25 to 0·5 mg by subcutaneous injection.

carbamazepine. An anticonvulsant effective in psychomotor epilepsy and grand mal, often in association with other drugs. Also effective in trigeminal neuralgia. Care is necessary in hepatic disease and glaucoma. Dose in epilepsy 200 to 1,200 mg daily, in neuralgia 100 mg or more.

carbarsone. An organic arsenic compound used in the treatment of amoebiasis. Dose 250 mg twice a day for ten days, often in association with emetine. The course may be repeated after a rest period of 4 to 7 days. Skin rash, urticaria and gastritis are occasional side-effects.

carbenicillin. A derivative of penicillin with a wider range of activity. Of great value in systemic and urinary infections due to *Pseudomonas aeruginosa* (*pyocyanea*), *Proteus*, and mixed infections. In severe systemic infections, large doses of 20 to 30 g daily by intravenous injection are given; for urinary infections, 1 to 2 g six-hourly by intramuscular injection.

carbenoxolone. A derivative of glycirrhiza, with anti-inflammatory properties resembling those of cortisone. Used in the treatment of gastric and duodenal ulcer, and locally for mouth ulcers. Side-effects include oedema and heartburn, and potassium supplements should be given to prevent hypokalaemia. Dose 50 to 100 mg.

carbimazole. An antithyroid drug. It inhibits the formation of thyroxine, *q.v.*, and is valuable for the oral treatment of thyrotoxicosis. May cause gastric disturbance in the early stages of treatment, but the drug may also cause fever and occasionally aplastic anaemia. Initial doses 30 to 60 mg daily; maintenance doses 5 to 20 mg daily.

Carbocaine. Mepivacaine, *q.v.*

carbolic acid. Phenol, *q.v.*

carbon dioxide. A colourless, non-inflammable gas. It has a stimulating effect on the respiratory centre, and a mixture of 5% of carbon dioxide in oxygen is used for respiratory depression. Solid carbon dioxide is used to destroy warts, naevi, etc.

Cardophylin. Aminophylline, *q.v.*

cascara. Has mild purgative properties. Dose: dry extract 100 to 250 mg, liquid extract and elixir, 2 to 5 ml.

castor oil. A mild purgative, often useful after food poisoning. Dose 5 to 20 ml. The oil has emollient properties, and is used together with zinc ointment for pressure sores, and napkin rash.

Catapres. Clonidine, *q.v.*

catechu. A plant extract used with chalk and other astringents in the treatment of diarrhoea. Dose of tincture of catechu 2 to 4 ml.

Cedilanid. Lanatoside C, *q.v.*

cefazolin (cephazolin). An antibiotic with general properties of the cephaloridines. Given by intramuscular injection in doses of 500 mg two to four times a day in respiratory and genito-urinary infections.

Celbenin. Methicillin, *q.v.*

Celontin. Methsuximide, *q.v.*

cephalexin. An antibiotic similar in action and uses to cephaloridine, *q.v.*, but active orally. Used mainly in respiratory and urinary tract infections. May cause nausea and diarrhoea. Dose 250 to 500 mg six-hourly.

cephaloridine. A bactericidal antibiotic effective against a wide range of organisms, including penicillin-resistant staphylococci, but not *Pseudomonas*. Of value in respiratory and urinary tract infections. Dose 0·5 to 1·5 g by intramuscular injection two or three times a day.

cephalothin. An antibiotic similar in action, uses and dose to cephaloridine, *q.v.* Often preferred if renal damage or dysfunction is present.

cephradine. An orally active antibiotic similar in action and dose to cephalexin, *q.v.*

Ceporex. Cephalexin, *q.v.*

Ceporin. Cephaloridine, *q.v.*

Cerubidin. Daunorubicin, *q.v.*

Cetiprin. Emepronium, *q.v.*

cetrimide. A detergent with antiseptic properties. Not effective against *Pseudomonas*, and only sterilized solutions should be used. The standard solution (1%) is suitable for wounds, burns, skin preparation and the removal of scabs.

chalk (calcium carbonate). An antacid used in alkaline preparations for the treatment of peptic ulcer. Also given with astringents such as catechu in the treatment of diarrhoea. Dose 1 to 4 g.

charcoal. A powerful adsorbent, given orally to remove intestinal gases in flatulence, and to mark the passage of faeces. Large doses may be given as a first-aid measure in poisoning by strychnine and many other toxic substances. Dose 4 to 8 g.

chiniofon. A derivative of iodoquinoline occasionally used in intestinal amoebiasis to supplement emetine therapy. Dose 0·2 to 1 g.

chloral hydrate. A water-soluble hypnotic with a prompt action. Of value for children and elderly patients who do not tolerate barbiturates. The drug must be given well diluted to reduce the gastric irritant effects. Dose 0·3 to 2 g.

chlorambucil. A cytostatic drug used in the treatment of malignant lymphoma and chronic lymphocytic leukaemia. It is relatively well tolerated, but strict haematological control of therapy is essential. Dose

0·2 mg per kg body-weight daily.

chloramphenicol. An orally active antibiotic. It has a wide range of activity, but is used mainly in typhoid and paratyphoid fevers. Prolonged or repeated treatment should be avoided, as severe damage to the blood-forming system may occur. It is also effective in intestinal and urinary infections, in whooping cough, and in many rickettsial and viral infections, but for these purposes less toxic drugs are now used. Chloramphenicol is also useful in skin and eye infections, and in otitis media. Average adult dose 500 mg four times a day, increased in severe infections. Children's doses range from 25 to 50 mg per kg body-weight daily; but the drug may be dangerous for infants.

chlorcyclizine. An antihistamine with a prolonged action. Drowsiness and other side-effects, such as dryness of the mouth, are uncommon. Dose 50 to 100 mg.

chlordiazepoxide. A psychotherapeutic drug with tranquillizing and muscle-relaxant properties. Widely used in the treatment of anxiety, tension, depression accompanied by agitation, and in alcoholism. Also useful in spastic neuromuscular disorders. The drug has a very wide margin of safety, and serious toxic effects are rare. Has been used by injection as a relaxant in tetanus. Dose 5 to 25 mg orally, 50 to 100 mg by injection.

chlorhexidine. An antiseptic of high potency and a wide range of activity, although it is ineffective against spores and viruses. Stock solutions of chlorhexidine and other antiseptics may become contaminated with *Pseudomonas*, and all such solutions should be freshly prepared. It is well tolerated by the tissues. For skin preparation a 0·5% solution in methylated spirit is used, but for general use a mixture of chlorhexidine with cetrimide (Savlon) is often preferred. A general-purpose cream and an obstetric cream are also available.

chlormethiazole. A sedative with anticonvulsant properties. Used by slow intravenous injection in acute mania, status epilepticus and toxaemia of pregnancy, and orally in alcoholism, epilepsy and insomnia. Oral dose 2 to 6 g daily.

chlorocresol. A disinfectant of high potency and low toxicity. It is used as a bactericide for injections in multiple-dose containers and in eye-drops.

chloroform. Once widely used as a general inhalation anaesthetic, but less toxic drugs are now preferred. Also used as chloroform water in mixtures as a preservative and flavouring agent, and for its carminative effects.

Chloromycetin. Chloramphenicol, *q.v.*

chloroquine. An anti-malarial drug effective against the erythrocytic forms of malarial parasites found in the blood, and used both for the suppression and treatment of malaria. Suppressive dose 0·3 g weekly. Treatment 0·6 g initially, followed by 0·3 g six to eight hours later, then 0·3 g daily for two days.

chlorothiazide. The first of the widely used group of thiazide diuretics. These drugs have a marked salt and water-eliminating action and are highly effective and well tolerated. Occasional side-effects include allergy and nausea. Chlorothiazide and related compounds are used extensively in congestive heart failure, and oedematous states generally. They are also used in hypertension, as they increase the activity of many hypotensive drugs and permit lower doses and reduce side-effects. Some potassium as well as sodium loss is caused by these drugs, and potassium chloride should be given to offset such loss if treatment is prolonged. Dose of chlorothiazide 0·5 to 2 g on alternate days.

chlorotrianisene. A synthetic oestrogen with a slow but prolonged action, and reduced side-effects such as nausea. Used in menopausal conditions; for the suppression of lactation, and in prostatic carcinoma. Dose 12 to 48 mg daily.

chloroxylenol. A non-irritating germicide, widely used in many non-caustic antiseptics. Although effective against streptococci, it is less active against staphylococci, and of little value against *Ps. pyocyanea* and *Proteus*.

chlorpheniramine. An antihistamine effective in oral doses of 4 to 16 mg daily. Also of value in the treatment of transfusion reactions and doses of 10 mg may be added to the intravenous drip solution.

chlorpromazine. A synthetic drug with a wide range of activity on the central nervous system. It is widely employed as an anti-emetic in nausea and vomiting; for potentiating the action of analgesics and hypnotics; for its powerful tranquillizing action in the treatment of agitation, tension and other psychiatric conditions; and the management of refractory and schizo-phrenic patients. Oral dose 25 to 50 mg, increased in mental disorders. Similar doses may be given by intravenous or deep intramuscular injection. It should not be given subcutaneously. It may cause obstructive jaundice in some patients, and blood dyscrasia may also occur. Care should be taken in handling any solution of the drug, as skin sensitization may occur after contact.

chlorpropamide. An oral hypoglycaemic agent of the tolbutamide type, *q.v.* It is used in the treatment of mild diabetes mellitus occurring in middle-aged patients. The drug is sometimes effective in patients who do not respond to tolbutamide, and in other cases may permit the insulin requirements to be reduced. Side-effects include rash, jaundice and blood dyscrasia, but are uncommon with low doses. Dose 250 to 500 mg daily as a single morning dose.

chlorprothixene. A tranquillizer related chemically to the chlorpromazine group of drugs, and used for similar purposes. Of value in acute conditions, less suitable for maintenance therapy. Dose 30 to 600 mg daily.

chlortetracycline. An orally effective antibiotic with the general properties of tetracyclines, q.v. Side-effects include stomatitis, diarrhoea, nausea; but these may be reduced by giving an antacid. Chlortetracycline may be given intravenously in emergency, but solutions must be injected very slowly, as vein inflammation may occur. Dose: oral, 250 mg six-hourly; intravenously, 100 to 500 mg.

chlorthalidone. A diuretic similar in action and uses to hydrochlorothiazide, q.v. Dose 100 to 200 mg daily.

Choledyl. A derivative of theophylline, q.v., with reduced gastric irritant effects.

chorionic gonadotrophin. A gonad-stimulating hormone derived from the placenta. It is used in metropathia haemorrhagica, habitual abortion, and undescended testicle. Dose 500 to 1,000 units by intramuscular injection.

Ciba 1906. Thiambutosine, q.v.

Cidomycin. Gentamicin, q.v.

cinchocaine. A local anaesthetic of high potency. Has been used for surface infiltration and spinal and urethral anaesthesia. Ointment, cream and suppositories are available.

cinnarizine. An antihistamine chiefly of value in Ménière's disease and motion sickness. Dose 45 to 90 mg daily.

clemastine. An antihistamine used in allergic rhinitis, urticaria and allergic dermatoses.

Dose 1 mg twice a day, up to a maximum of 6 mg daily.

clindamycin. An antibiotic with actions and uses similar to lincomycin, q.v. Dose 150 to 450 mg six-hourly.

clobetasone. A topically active steroid of use in a wide range of inflammatory skin conditions. Absorption with systemic effects may occur if applied extensively.

clofazimine. An antileprotic agent, of value in conditions resistant to dapsone, q.v. May cause discoloration of the skin and lesions. Dose 100 mg three to six times a week.

clofibrate. A drug which lowers the level of cholesterol and triglycerides in the blood, and so of value in atherosclerosis. May potentiate the action of anticoagulants, the dose of which should be reduced during clofibrate treatment. Not advised during pregnancy. Dose 20 mg per kg body-weight up to 2 g daily.

clomocycline. A derivative of tetracycline, with a similar range of anti-bacterial activity; but absorbed and excreted more rapidly, and effective in the lower dose of 170 mg six-hourly.

clonidine. A potent drug used in the treatment of hypertension, especially when guanethidine is not tolerated. Dose

75 micrograms initially, increased slowly to a daily dose of 1 mg or more. In doses of 50 micrograms daily, it is used in the prophylactic treatment of migraine.

clopamide. A diuretic with an action similar to chlorothiazide, but with a more rapid and reliable effect. Dose 20 to 60 mg daily, or as necessary, taken at morning to avoid nocturia. As with other diuretics, some potassium loss may occur. Clopamide also has some hypotensive properties.

cloxacillin. A semi-synthetic derivative of penicillin that, unlike the parent drug, is not broken down by the enzyme penicillinase, and so is effective against resistant staphylococci. Oral adult dose is 500 mg six-hourly; in severe infections cloxacillin may be given by intramuscular or intravenous injection in doses of 250 to 500 mg six-hourly.

coal tar. The black viscous liquid obtained from the distillation of coal. It is used mainly as Zinc and Tar Paste in eczema, psoriasis and pruritus.

cocaine. A powerful local anaesthetic, but it has been largely replaced by less toxic synthetic compounds. Used in ophthalmology as a 2% solution, often with homatropine, *q.v.*

cod-liver oil. A rich source of vitamins A and D. It is used as a dietary supplement to improve general nutrition, promote calcification and prevent rickets. Dose 2 to 10 ml daily.

codeine. One of the alkaloids of opium. It depresses the cough centre and is widely prescribed for the treatment of useless cough. It also has mild analgesic properties, and is used with aspirin in Compound Codeine Tablets and similar preparations. In large doses the constipating action of codeine may be a disadvantage. Dose 10 to 60 mg.

Cogentin. Benztropine, *q.v.*

colaspase. An enzyme that breaks down the amino-acid asparagine, which is essential for the development of some malignant cells. Colaspase has an indirect effect on the growth of such cells. Used mainly in acute leukaemia. Dose 200 units per kg bodyweight daily by slow intravenous injection.

colchicum. The dried corm of meadow saffron. It contains the alkaloid colchicine, which is used for the relief of acute gout, and is given in doses of 0·5 mg every two hours until relief is obtained. A total dose of 6 mg should not be exceeded, but relief of pain or the onset of vomiting or purging usually renders full doses unnecessary.

colistin. An antibiotic chiefly effective against Gram-negative organisms, and given orally in gastro-enteritis. For systemic and urinary infections it must be given by intramuscular or intravenous injection in doses of 3 to 9 mega units daily. Resistance to colistin is uncommon. Side-effects after injection include mild neurotoxic disturbances, and more rarely nephrotoxic symptoms.

collodion. A solution of pyroxylin used as a protective dressing to small wounds.

Colomycin. Colistin, *q.v.*

Concordin. Protriptyline, *q.v.*

congo red. A red dye used by intravenous injection as a 1% solution in the diagnosis of amyloid disease. The degree of absorption of the dye from the blood one hour after injection is measured, and a loss of more than 30% is an indication of amyloid disease.

copper sulphate. Blue crystals soluble in water. The main constituent of Clinitest tablets and Benedict's solution used for testing for glucose in urine.

Coramine. Nikethamide, *q.v.*

corticotrophin. The adrenocorticotrophic hormone of the anterior pituitary gland. It stimulates the production of corticoid hormones by the adrenal cortex, especially hydrocortisone, and hence has a wide range of activity. The drug has a rapid action and is very useful in the treatment of severe asthma and allergic states and in some inflammatory conditions. It is not effective in adrenal deficiency states, where replacement therapy with cortisone is necessary. The dose varies from 10–25 units four times a day by intramuscular or subcutaneous injection, but long-acting forms are also available. The effects are often dramatic but transient, and symptoms may return if the drug is withdrawn too quickly. The side-effects are due to pituitary imbalance, and may include Cushing's syndrome, water and salt retention, mental disturbances, and the reactivation of peptic ulcers and tuberculous lesions.

cortisone. One of the most important of the steroid hormones secreted by the adrenal cortex. Together with hydrocortisone, it plays a major part in the body metabolism, controlling the formation of glucose, the salt and water balance, the resistance to stress, and the response to inflammatory and allergic stimuli. Corticosteroids are also of value in leukaemia and other blood disorders, and as immunosuppressive agents in transplant surgery. Cortisone is used mainly in Addisons' disease and related conditions, where its salt-retaining action is an advantage. In other systemic inflammatory conditions, such as rheumatoid arthritis, this salt-retaining action is undesirable, and many alternative drugs such as prednisone, triamcinolone and betamethasone have been introduced which have a more specific action. Dose of cortisone 25 mg orally, or by intramuscular injection, based upon need and response, later slowly reduced or eventually withdrawn. For topical use in many inflamed skin conditions, hydrocortisone, beclomethasone or fluocinolone are preferred. These steroids have no antibacterial action, and for infected conditions, hydrocortisone and related drugs are often used in association with neomycin, q.v.

Cosmegen. Actinomycin D, q.v.

Crasnitin. Colaspase, q.v.

cresol. A powerful antiseptic similar to phenol. It is the principal constituent of lysol, q.v.

crystal violet. A dyestuff with a selective antiseptic action against Gram-positive organisms and yeasts. Used as a 0·5% solution for burns, boils and carbuncles, and an alcoholic solution with brilliant green is used for skin preparation.

Crystamycin. A mixture of penicillin and streptomycin. Effective against a wide range of common infections.

Cuprimine. Penicillamine, q.v.

cyanocobalamin. The antianaemic factor present in liver. It is specific in the treatment of pernicious anaemia, and its neurological complications, and of value in other macrocytic anaemias due to nutritional deficiencies. In large doses it has been used for the relief of certain neurological conditions such as herpes zoster. Dose in pernicious anaemia 1,000 micrograms or more, once or twice weekly by intramuscular injection. Maintenance doses of 250 micrograms can be given at longer intervals. Cyanocobalamin is rapidly excreted, and for maintenance hydroxocobalamin, q.v., is often preferred.

cyclobarbitone. A short-acting barbiturate with the general sedative effects of that group of drugs. Dose 200 to 400 mg.

cyclopenthiazide. One of the thiazide group of diuretics. Effective in many oedematous conditions, and also in hypertension as an adjuvant to other hypotensive drugs. Dose 1 mg initially, 250 to 500 micrograms daily as necessary.

cyclophosphamide. A cytostatic drug, active orally and by injection, with an action similar to mustine. Used in Hodgkin's disease and other cancerous conditions. Dose 50 to 200 mg orally, 100 to 200 mg intravenously.

cyclopropane. An inhalation anaesthetic of high potency with which induction and recovery are rapid. It causes some respiratory depression and cardiac irregularities, and its administration requires care. It is used with closed-circuit apparatus. Supplied in orange-coloured cylinders.

cycloserine. An antibiotic active chiefly against the tubercle bacillus, and used in severe pulmonary tuberculosis when standard drugs are ineffective. Occasionally used in urinary infections. Dose 250 to 750 mg daily.

cyproheptadine. A powerful antihistamine and antiserotonin compound. Some allergic reactions are due not only to histamine, but also to serotonin, and cyproheptadine is useful in conditions not responding completely to an antihistamine. Dose 4 mg.

Cytamen. Cyanocobalamin, *q.v.*

cytarabine. A cytostatic agent that prevents cell development by inhibiting the formation of nucleic acid. May induce remission in acute leukaemia. Dose 3 mg per kg body-weight daily by intravenous injection, according to response.

Cytosar. Cytarabine, *q.v.*

D

DADPS. Dapsone, *q.v.*

D.D.T. Dicophane, *q.v.*

D.F. 118. Dihydrocodeine bitartrate. A derivative of codeine with a more powerful analgesic action. Useful when an analgesic is required without resorting to morphine or other opiate. Dose 30 to 60 mg orally; 50 mg by injection.

D.O.C.A. Deoxycortone acetate, *q.v.*

Dalacin C. Clindamycin, *q.v.*

Dalmane. Flurazepam, *q.v.*

danazol. A derivative of ethisterone that inhibits the release of pituitary gonadotrophins. Used in conditions where such release is necessary, as in endometriosis and precocious puberty. Care is necessary in cardiac, renal and hepatic dysfunction. Dose 100 to 800 mg daily.

Dantrium. Dantrolene, *q.v.*

dantrolene. A skeletal muscle-relaxant that appears to act within the muscle fibre, and not at the myoneural junction. Used in severe spastic states following stroke and spinal cord injury. Dose 25 mg initially, increasing to 400 mg daily as required. May cause hepatotoxicity, and its use needs care.

Daonil. Glibenclamide, q.v.

dapsone. A sulphone compound used in the treatment of lepromatous and tuberculoid leprosy and in dermatitis herpetiformis. Dose: orally, 25 to 100 mg twice weekly in leprosy; daily doses of 50 to 200 mg in dermatitis herpetiformis.

Daranide. Dichlorphenamide, q.v.

Daraprim. Pyrimethamine, q.v.

Dartalan. Thiopropazate, q.v.

daunorubicin. An antibiotic with cytostatic properties, used in lymphoblastic and myeloblastic leukaemia. Given intravenously in controlled doses of 0·5 to 3 mg.

debrisoquine. A well-tolerated hypotensive drug effective in all types of hypertension, including those not responding to other drugs. It lowers the blood pressure by decreasing peripheral resistance. initial dose 20 mg, increasing by 10 mg to maintenance doses of 40 to 120 mg daily.

Side-effects may be reduced by combined treatment with a thiazide diuretic.

Decadron. Dexamethasone, q.v.

Declinax. Debrisoquine, q.v.

Degranol. Mannomustine, q.v.

deoxycortone. One of the principal hormones of the cortex of the adrenal gland, controlling sodium retention and potassium excretion. Once widely used in the treatment of Addison's disease, but now occasionally employed to supplement cortisone therapy. Dose 2 to 10 mg by intramuscular injection.

Depixol. Flupenthixol, q.v.

Depostat. Gestronol, q.v.

Deseril. Methysergide, q.v.

Desferal. Desferrioxamine, q.v.

desferrioxamine. A substance that combines with iron salts to form a soluble non-toxic complex. Of great value in acute iron poisoning in children in a dose of 2 g immediately by intramuscular injection, together with 5 g orally.

desipramine. A derivative of imipramine, q.v., with similar antidepressant properties, but with a more rapid action. A response may be apparent within a week of treatment. Dose: 25 to 75 mg, increasing to 200 mg daily orally, 25 to 50 mg by intramuscular injection.

dexamethasone. A synthetic corticosteroid with reduced

salt-retaining properties. Useful in all conditions requiring glucocorticoid therapy except Addison's disease. Dose 0·5 to 10 mg daily.

dexamphetamine sulphate. A central nervous system stimulant similar to amphetamine, *q.v.*; but it also has appetite-depressant properties, and has been used in the treatment of obesity. Dose 5 to 10 mg.

Dexedrine. Dexamphetamine sulphate, *q.v.*

dextran. A blood-plasma substitute obtained from sucrose solutions by bacterial action. Of value in burns, shock, etc., when blood or plasma is not available. Special dextran solutions are used to reduce blood viscosity and red cell aggregation, and to improve peripheral circulation.

dextromoramide. A synthetic morphine-like analgesic of value in severe and intractable pain. Dose 5 mg or more either orally or by injection, according to need and response.

dextropropoxyphene. A potent orally effective analgesic. Of value in many painful conditions, and in malignant disease, its use may delay the need to resort to the opiate analgesics. Dose 30 to 60 mg.

dextrose. A readily absorbed carbohydrate found in many sweet fruits, but obtained commercially by the hydrolysis of starch. It is given orally as a dietary supplement; in acidosis; and to raise the glycogen reserve of the liver in poisoning by drugs causing hepatic damage. Given by intravenous injection as a 5% solution or as dextrose-saline in severe dehydration, shock, and after abdominal operations until fluids can again be taken orally.

Diaginol. Sodium acetrizoate, *q.v.*

Diabinese. Chlorpropamide, *q.v.*

diamorphine. A derivative of morphine with a more powerful analgesic and cough-suppressant action. Valuable for the relief of severe pain and the suppression of useless cough. Addiction is a constant risk owing to the euphoric effects of the drug, and the use of diamorphine, except in terminal cases, has declined as more satisfactory morphine-like analgesics have become available. Dose 5 to 10 mg or more as required.

Diamox. Acetazolamide, *q.v.*

Dianabol. Methandienone, *q.v.*

diazepam. A tranquillizing drug similar to chlordiazepoxide, *q.v.*, and of value in anxiety and agitated-depressive states. It also has muscle-relaxant and tension-relieving properties, and is useful for pre-medication as well as psychiatric states. Dose 4 to 40 mg daily.

diazoxide. An inhibitor of insulin secretion. Used intravenously in severe hypoglycaemia in doses of 2 to 5 mg per kg body-weight. Also of value in severe hypertensive crisis in doses of 300 mg by rapid intravenous injection.

Dibenyline. Phenoxybenzamine, *q.v.*

Dibotin. Phenformin, *q.v.*

dichlorophen. A powerful anthelmintic effective against the beef tapeworm. Unlike other anti-tapeworm drugs, which loosen the hold of the parasites, dichlorophen kills the worms, which are then excreted in a semi-digested state. Previous fasting and subsequent purgation are unnecessary. Dose: 6 g daily for two days, children may be given two doses of 2 to 4 g. Colic and vomiting are side-effects.

dichlorphenamide. An inhibitor of carbonic anhydrase. Used in glaucoma, and in the chronic respiratory insufficiency of acute bronchitis. Dose 25 to 50 mg. Long-term treatment may cause electrolyte disturbance.

dicophane (D.D.T.). An effective but slow-acting contact insecticide; valuable in the elimination of body parasites

as dicophane application (2%), or dusting powder (10%).

dicyclomine. A synthetic atropine-like compound, used to reduce hyperacidity and for its antispasmodic action in peptic ulcer, biliary spasm, colic and pylorospasm. Dose 10 to 20 mg.

Dicynene. Ethamsylate, *q.v.*

dienoestrol. Synthetic oestrogen similar to stilboestrol, but less active. Dose 1 to 10 mg.

diethylcarbamazine. A synthetic drug used in filariasis. Effective chiefly against microfilariae, and thus reduces spread of the disease by insects. Longer treatment is necessary to kill the adult worms. Dose 150 to 500 mg daily. Low initial doses may be necessary to reduce allergic reactions due to proteins released from dead worms.

diethylpropion. An appetite depressant related chemically to the amphetamines, but with reduced central stimulant effects. Dose 25 mg.

Digitaline Nativelle. Preparations of digitoxin *q.v.* Tablets or granules of 0·1 mg and 0·25 mg, oral solution 1:1,000, ampoules 0·2 mg for intramuscular injection.

digitalis. The leaf of the common foxglove. A powerful cardiac tonic, slowing, strengthening and regulating the action of the heart. It is used in congestive heart failure, atrial fibrillation and flutter. The diuretic effects are secondary and are due to the improvement in the general circulation. The drug is eliminated slowly, and nausea and vomiting are usually signs that the dosage should be reduced. Dose of digitalis leaf, 100 to 200 mg, often in association with diuretics. Elderly patients may require smaller doses. Large initial doses of 1 g or more are occasionally used, but for massive emergency doses, digoxin, q.v., is now preferred.

digitoxin. The most powerful cardiac glycoside of digitalis leaf. Absorption is rapid but excretion is slow, and cumulative effects may occur. Maintenance dose 0·05 to 0·2 mg daily, but larger doses may be given initially.

digoxin. A powerful cardiac glycoside from the Austrian foxglove *Digitalis lanata*. It is more rapidly absorbed and excreted than digitalis leaf, so the effect is more prompt and easily controlled. One tablet (0·25 mg) is equivalent to about 60 mg of digitalis leaf. Dose 1 to 1·5 mg initially, followed by maintenance doses of 0·25 mg once or twice daily. Elderly patients and children require smaller doses and a special tablet containing 0·0625 mg is available. For rapid digitalization in congestive heart failure or fibrillation, a dose of 0·5 to 1 mg may be given by intramuscular or slow intravenous injection.

dihydrotachysterol. A.T.10, *q.v.*

di-iodohydroxyquinoline. Used orally in chronic intestinal amoebiasis and amoebic dysentery, chiefly as a supplement to emetine. Dose 1 to 2 g daily in divided doses for 20 days. Intestinal disturbances and, rarely, optic neuritis may occur. Also used as pessaries (100 mg) in trichomonal infections.

diloxanide. A synthetic amoebicide used mainly in the treatment of intestinal amoebiasis, either alone or to supplement emetine treatment. Dose 1·5 g daily for 10 days.

Dimelor. Acetohexamide, *q.v.*

dimenhydrinate. An anti-emetic drug similar to some antihistamines. Used mainly to prevent travel sickness, vomiting of pregnancy, and radiation sickness. Dose 50 mg.

dimercaprol (B.A.L.). A clear liquid, used in the treatment of poisoning by arsenic, mercury and gold. Early treatment is essential in mercury poisoning to prevent kidney damage. Given by intramuscular injection as 5% solution in arachis oil. Dose 8 to 16 ml in divided doses for one day, subsequent doses of 2 to 4 ml daily according to need.

Dindevan. Phenindione, *q.v.*

dinoprostone. A synthetic form of prostaglandin E$_2$. It initiates contractions of the pregnant uterus, and has been used orally and intravenously in doses of 0·5 mg to initiate labour. Larger doses have been given to terminate pregnancy. Its availability is restricted to approved centres.

diodone injection. A solution of a complex organic iodine compound, used as a contrast agent in X-ray examination of kidneys and ureters. Stronger solutions are used in angiocardiography, etc. Dose 20 ml intravenously.

Diodoquin. Di-iodohydroxyquinoline, *q.v.*

diphenhydramine. One of the early antihistamines. Used in the treatment of allergic conditions, including urticaria, rhinitis, atopic dermatitis, hay-fever, and drug reactions. It also has a sedative action, which in some allergic conditions is an advantage. Also useful in travel sickness. Dose 50 to 200 mg daily.

Dipidolor. Piritamide, *q.v.*

Disipal. Orphenadrine, *q.v.*

Di-Sipidin. Pituitary extract in powder form for use as a snuff in diabetes insipidus and enuresis. Careful application

of the snuff is essential to obtain the maximum effects.

disopyramide. An anticholinergic drug used in the oral treatment of cardiac arrhythmias. The dose varies from 300 to 800 mg daily according to need. Care is necessary if a degree of heart block is present, and by its anticholinergic action, glaucoma and urinary retention can be contra-indications.

Distamine. Penicillamine, *q.v.*

distigmine. An inhibitor of cholinesterase similar to neostigmine, *q.v.*, but used mainly in the treatment of neurogenic bladder, and the postoperative retention of urine. Occasionally used in myasthenia gravis as an alternative to other drugs. Dose 5 mg orally, 500 micrograms by intramuscular injection.

disulfiram. Tetraethylthiuram disulphide. When taken in association with alcohol, side-effects such as flushing, giddiness, vomiting and headache occur. The drug has therefore been used in chronic alcoholism, but prolonged treatment and co-operation of the patient are essential. Dose 200 to 400 mg daily.

dithranol. Synthetic compound used mainly in the treatment of psoriasis. The drug is a powerful irritant, and treatment should be commenced with a simple ointment or zinc paste containing 0·1%, gradually increased to 1% if well tolerated.

Dixarit. Clonidine, *q.v.* for the prophylactic treatment of migraine.

Doloxene. Dextropropoxyphene, *q.v.*

domiphen bromide. A detergent antiseptic with a range of activity similar to cetrimide, *q.v.* Lozenges for throat infections are available.

Dopram. Doxapram, *q.v.*

Doriden. Glutethimide, *q.v.*

Dover's powder. Contains ipecacuanha and opium. Once widely used as a diaphoretic. Dose 0·3 to 0·6 g.

doxapram. A respiratory stimulant useful in post-operative depression, or that caused by narcotic analgesics. Dose, by intravenous infusion, 0·5 to 4 mg per minute.

doxepin. An antidepressant of the imipramine type, but with additional tranquillizing properties. Used in the treatment of depression accompanied by anxiety. Dose 30 to 300 mg daily.

doxorubicin. An antibiotic with cytostatic properties. Used in leukaemia and lymphosarcoma. Toxic effects may limit treatment. Dose 0·5 mg per kg body-weight daily by intravenous injection.

doxycycline. A tetracycline

derivative characterized by a high degree of absorption and a slow rate of excretion. Following an initial dose of 200 mg an adequate blood-level can be maintained by a single daily dose of 100 mg.

Dramamine. Dimenhydrinate, *q.v.*

Droleptan. Droperidol, *q.v.*

Dromoran. Levorphanol, *q.v.*

droperidol. A tranquilliser with unusual properties. Used mainly with analgesics to produce a state of detachment before various diagnostic procedures.

drostanolone. A synthetic compound with some of the anabolic and androgenic properties of testosterone. Of value in the treatment of carcinoma of the breast in doses of 100 mg once to three times a week by intramuscular injection.

Dulcolax. Bisacodyl, *q.v.*

Duogastrone. Carbenoxolone, *q.v.*, in a capsule for the treatment of duodenal ulcer.

Duphalac. Lactulose, *q.v.*

Duphaston. Dydrogesterone, *q.v.*

Durabolin. Nandrolone, *q.v.*

dydrogesterone. A progesterone-like compound used mainly in threatened abortion and to promote fertility. Also useful in dysmenorrhoea. Dose 10 to 20 mg.

Dytac. Triamterene, *q.v.*

E

E.B.I. Emetine bismuth iodide.

Edecrin. Ethacrynic acid, *q.v.*

Eltroxin. Thyroxine, *q.v.*

emepronium. A compound with an atropine-like action on the muscular tone of the urinary bladder. Useful in urinary frequency and tenesmus. Dose 50 to 100 mg.

Emeside. Ethosuximide, *q.v.*

emetine. An alkaloid obtained from ipecacuanha, and used in the treatment of acute amoebic dysentery, usually in combination with other amoebicides to obtain maximum effect. Dose 30 to 60 mg daily by subcutaneous or intramuscular injection. Also of value in amoebic abscess. For oral use emetine bismuth iodide is preferred as with that compound the emetic side-effects of emetine are reduced. Dose 60 to 200 mg daily.

Endoxana. Cyclophosphamide, *q.v.*

Enduron. Methylclothiazide, *q.v.*

Envacar. Guanoxan, *q.v.*

Epanutin. Phenytoin sodium, *q.v.*

ephedrine. A sympathomimetic agent, with a marked relaxant effect on the bronchioles, valuable in the treatment of asthma and bronchial spasm. It also constricts the peripheral vessels, and has been used to counteract the fall in blood-pressure that may occur during general and spinal anaesthesia. Occasionally used in whooping cough, enuresis and as a mydriatic. Care is necessary in hypertension and prostatic enlargement. Dose 15 to 60 mg.

Ephynal. Tocopherol, *q.v.*

Epilim. Sodium valproate, *q.v.*

epinephrine. Adrenaline, *q.v.*

Epontol. Propanidid, *q.v.*

Eppy. A non-irritant solution of adrenaline, *q.v.*, used as eye-drops to reduce intra-ocular pressure in glaucoma.

Epsikapron. Aminocaproic acid, *q.v.*

Eptoin. Phenytoin sodium, *q.v.*

Equanil. Meprobamate, *q.v.*

ergometrine. The principal alkaloid of ergot, *q.v.* It promotes uterine contraction but is mainly used to control post-partum haemorrhage. Dangerous in the early stages of labour. Dose 0·5 to 1 mg orally, or by intramuscular injection, smaller doses intravenously.

ergot. A fungus that develops in the ovary of rye and replaces the normal grain. The active principles include ergometrine, *q.v.*, and ergotamine, *q.v.* Chronic toxic effects characterized by gangrene of the extremities, have followed the use of ergot-containing rye bread.

ergotamine tartrate. One of the

alkaloids of ergot, *q.v.* Has some oxytocic effects but therapeutically it is used almost entirely for the relief of migraine. Early dosage produces the best effects, but it should not be used prophylactically owing to the risk of ergotism. Dose 1 to 2 mg orally, up to a total of 6 mg; 0·25 to 0·5 mg by subcutaneous injection. It may also be given by oral inhalation.

erythrityl tetranitrate. A vasodilator similar to glyceryl trinitrate, *q.v.*, but with a less intense and more prolonged action. Dose 15 to 60 mg.

erythromycin. An orally effective antibiotic, resembling penicillin in its range of activity. Useful in acute streptococcal infections, in pneumonia, and staphylococcal enteritis. It is inactivated by gastric acid, and should be given as coated tablets, or as a suspension of more stable derivatives. In severe infections it may be given by intravenous or intramuscular injection. Dose 250 mg.

Esbatal. Bethanidine, *q.v.*

eserine. Physostigmine, *q.v.*

Esidrex. Hydrochlorothiazide, *q.v.* Esidrex-K contains added potassium chloride, to offset the potassium loss in the urine which may occur when treatment is prolonged.

Eskacef. Cephradine, *q.v.*

ethacrynic acid. A powerful diuretic with a rapid and intense action. It may be effective when the response to thiazide diuretics is inadequate. Maintenance treatment needs care, as loss of salts and water is considerable, and potassium supplements may be necessary. Dose 50 mg daily in the mornings, increased by 25 mg daily as necessary up to 200 mg in divided doses.

ethambutol. An antitubercular drug, of value in patients hypersensitive or resistant to standard drugs. Dose 25 mg per kg body-weight daily, reduced after two months to 15 mg. It may cause visual disturbances, and lower doses should be given in renal damage.

ethamsylate. A systemically effective haemostatic agent used to control bleeding from small blood-vessels as in haematuria, or in surgery. Dose 500 mg orally, 250 mg by intravenous injection.

ether. A colourless inflammable liquid, once widely used as volatile general anaesthetic but replaced to a large extent by halothane, *q.v.* Induction of anaesthesia with ether is unpleasant, and thiopentone or nitrous oxide is often preferred for the first stage of anaesthesia.

ethinyloestradiol. A synthetic oestrogen more active than stilboestrol, *q.v.*, and with fewer side-effects. Used in menopausal symptoms, amenorrhoea, uterine hypoplasia, functional uterine bleeding, and other conditions where oestrogen therapy is indicated. It is present with a progestogen in many oral contraceptive products. Dose 0·01 to 0·1 mg daily. Larger doses are given in prostatic and mammary carcinoma.

ethionamide. An antitubercular drug useful in conditions resistant to other tuberculostatic drugs. Combined treatment is necessary, as bacterial resistance is soon acquired if ethionamide is used alone. Dose 500 mg to 1 g daily, but gastric disturbances are likely with the larger dose.

ethisterone. A synthetic progestogen similar in action to progesterone, but active orally. In amenorrhoea it may be given in association with an oestrogen. Dose 25 to 100 mg daily.

ethopropazine. A spasmolytic drug chemically related to the phenothiazine tranquillizers, but used mainly in the treatment of parkinsonism. It may cause more side-effects than associated drugs such as benzhexol. Reduces rigidity more than tremor. Dose 50 to 100 mg initially daily in divided doses, subsequently according to need and response to a maximum of 500 mg daily. May be used in association with atropine-like drugs for maximum effect, but transference from or to other drugs should be gradual.

ethosuximide. An anticonvulsant for the treatment of petit mal epilepsy. May be used alone, or combined with other anticonvulsants, and often of value in patients not responding to other drugs. Dose 250 mg daily initially, gradually increased if required to a maximum of 2 g daily.

ethotoin. An anticonvulsant sometimes used in epilepsy not responding to other drugs. Dose 2 g daily.

ethyl biscoumacetate. An oral anticoagulant used similarly to phenindione, *q.v.*, in the prophylaxis and treatment of thrombosis. Absorption is rapid, but when an immediate action is essential injections of heparin, *q.v.*, are also given. Nausea and alopecia are occasional side-effects. Initial dose 1·2 g; subsequent doses vary from 150 to 900 mg daily, and are based on prothrombin times.

ethyl chloride. A volatile anaesthetic used for induction or short operations only. It is a gas at ordinary temperatures, but is supplied in glass containers as a liquid. It is also a local anaesthetic by virtue of the intense cold produced by its evaporation.

Eudemine. Diazoxide, q.v.

Euglucon. Glibenclamide, q.v.

Eumydrin. Atropine methonitrate, q.v.

eusol. A chlorine antiseptic solution used as lotion, or as compress. The solution should be freshly prepared.

Eutonyl. Pargyline, q.v.

F

Fabahistin. Mebhydrolin, q.v.

Femergin. Ergotamine tartrate, q.v.

fenfluramine. An appetite depressant without the stimulant effects of related drugs. May cause diarrhoea with some patients. Dose 40 to 120 mg daily.

fenoprofen. A non-steroidal anti-inflammatory and antirheumatic agent. Useful as an alternative drug in rheumatoid arthritis and related conditions. Dose 250 mg twice a day.

Fenopron. Fenoprofen, q.v.

fentanyl. A morphine-like analgesic, used in association with tranquillizers such as droperidol, q.v., to produce a state of 'neurolepto-analgesia'.

Fentazin. Perphenazine, q.v.

ferrous gluconate, sulphate. These compounds are listed under iron, q.v.

Flagyl. Metronidazole, q.v.

flavoxate. An antispasmodic of value in urinary disorders such as cystitis, urethritis and related conditions. Dose 200 mg three times a day. Not recommended for children.

Flaxedil. Gallamine, q.v.

Florinef. Fludrocortisone, q.v.

Floxapen. Flucloxacillin, q.v.

flucloxacillin. A derivative of cloxacillin, q.v., but is absorbed more readily when given orally. Dose 250 mg six-hourly before meals. In severe infections it may be given by intramuscular or intravenous injection.

fludrocortisone. A synthetic steroid with a very powerful salt-retaining action. Valuable in adrenal deficiency state such as Addison's disease, usually to supplement cortisone treatment. Initial dose 1 to 2 mg, maintenance dose 0·1 to 0·2 mg daily.

flufenamic acid. An analgesic and anti-inflammatory drug of value in rheumatoid and arthritic conditions. May cause gastric disturbance which can be reduced by divided doses taken after food. Dose 400 to 600 mg daily. Use with care in renal disease and peptic ulcer. Contraindicated in pregnancy.

fluocinolone. A corticosteroid more active by topical application than hydrocortisone as an anti-inflammatory agent. Used as cream, ointment or lotion 0·01 to 0·025%; also with neomycin 0·5% in inflamed and infected skin conditions.

fluorescein. An orange-red compound, solutions of which have a strong green fluorescence. It is used as eye-drops (2%) for detecting corneal lesions, as areas of cornea denuded of epithelium stain green. Sometimes given by injection to facilitate examination of retinal blood-vessels.

Fluothane. Halothane, *q.v.*

flupenthixol. A tranquillizer similar to fluphenazine, and used in the depot treatment of schizophrenia. Dose 1 to 4 mg daily or 20 to 40 mg by deep intramuscular injection at intervals of 2 to 4 weeks.

fluphenazine. A phenothiazine derivative with more powerful tranquillizing and antiemetic properties than chlorpromazine. Dose 1 to 2 mg daily in anxiety states, up to 15 mg daily in schizophrenia. A long-acting form for intramuscular injection (25 mg) has an effect lasting 2 to 3 weeks.

flurazepam. A non-barbiturate hypnotic similar to nitrazepam, *q.v.* It is of low toxicity,

and the risk of 'hangover' effects is slight. Dose 15 to 30 mg.

fluspirilene. A long-acting major tranquillizer, used by intramuscular injection in schizophrenia. Dose 2 mg weekly initially, average maintenance doses 2 to 8 mg weekly. Care is necessary in epilepsy.

folic acid. A constituent of the vitamin B group. It is essential for cell division and the growth and development of normal red blood cells. The main use is in the treatment of nutritional macrocytic anaemias, pellagra and tropical sprue. Folic acid deficiency may occur in pregnancy, and small doses are present in many iron preparations to prevent the megaloblastic anaemia that may occur in later stages of pregnancy. It should not be used in pernicious anaemia, as it cannot prevent the degeneration of the central nervous system associated with that disease. Dose 5 to 20 mg; 0·2 to 0·5 mg for prophylaxis during pregnancy.

formaldehyde. A powerful but toxic germicide used mainly as 'formalin' in the disinfection of rooms; as a constituent of instrument storage solutions, and as 'formal-saline' (5% in normal saline) for the preservation of pathological specimens. Warts have been treated with a 3% solution.

formalin. A 40% solution of formaldehyde, *q.v.*

Fortral. Pentazocine, *q.v.*

fosfestrol. Has the general properties of stilboestrol, *q.v.*, but is used mainly in the treatment of carcinoma of the prostate. Given orally in doses of 100 mg or more thrice daily, or by intravenous injection.

framycetin. An antibiotic resembling neomycin, *q.v.*, in general properties. Used as cream, ointment and lotion. Given by subconjunctival injection in eye infections, and orally for gastro-intestinal infections. Dose 1 to 1·5 g.

Framygen. Framycetin, *q.v.*

French chalk. Talc, *q.v.*

friar's balsam. Contains benzoin, storax, aloes, balsam of tolu. Official name Compound Tincture of Benzoin. Used internally and by inhalation in bronchitis, etc., dose 2 to 4 ml.

frusemide. A diuretic with a powerful and intense action of short duration. Often effective in conditions no longer responding to thiazide diuretics. Dose 40 to 80 mg as a single dose, repeated three times a week, or 20 mg by intravenous injection. Larger doses may be necessary in acute renal failure. Nausea, diarrhoea and cramp may occur, and supplementary potassium is usually necessary.

Fucidin. Sodium fusidate, *q.v.*

Fulcin. Griseofulvin, *q.v.*

Fungilin. Amphotericin, *q.v.*

Furacin. Nitrofurazone, *q.v.*

Furadantin. Nitrofurantoin, *q.v.*

Furamide. Diloxanide, *q.v.*

G

gallamine triethiodide. A synthetic muscle relaxant with an action similar to that of tubocurarine, *q.v.*, but the effect is less prolonged. Is used extensively in surgery, as it is well tolerated, but pre-medication with atropine is necessary to avoid excessive salivation. Also used in convulsive shock therapy to reduce risk of injury. The action of the drug can be terminated by neostigmine. Average initial dose 80 to 120 mg, with small subsequent doses according to need and response.

Gammexane. Benzene hexachloride, an insecticide similar to D.D.T., but much more powerful and rapid, and less toxic.

Gantanol. Sulphamethoxazole, *q.v.*

Gantrisin. Sulphafurazole, *q.v.*

Gardenal. Phenobarbitone, *q.v.*

Gee's linctus. A soothing cough linctus containing camphorated tincture of opium, oxymel of squill and syrup of tolu. Dose 2 to 4 ml.

gelatin. Protein material used in nutrient jellies, and as gelatin-glycerin base for pessaries and suppositories.

gentamicin. An antibiotic effective against a wide range of organisms, including *Proteus* and *Pseudomonas*. Of value in Gram-negative infections, often in association with other drugs. Not absorbed orally, and for systemic infections is given by intramuscular injection in doses of 40 to 80 mg. Applied as cream, ointment or drops for local infections.

gentian violet. Crystal violet, *q.v.*

Genticin. Gentamicin, *q.v.*

gestronol. A synthetic oestrogen used in the treatment of endometrial carcinoma and benign prostatic hypertrophy. Dose 200 to 400 mg by intramuscular injection once a week.

glibenclamide. An orally active hypoglycaemic agent, basically similar to chlorpropamide, but effective in doses varying from 2·5 to 20 mg daily.

Glibenese. Glipizide, *q.v.*

glibornuride. An orally active hypoglycaemic agent used in late onset diabetes. It is more potent than many related drugs, and is given in doses of 25 to 50 mg daily at breakfast.

glipizide. A sulphonylurea, used like tolbutamide, *q.v.*, in diabetes, but effective in much lower doses. Initial dose 5 mg, maintenance doses 2.5 to 30 mg daily.

glucagon. A hormone of the pancreas which raises the blood sugar level by mobilizing liver glycogen. Used in insulin hypoglycaemia in doses of 0·5 to 1 mg by injection. Large doses by intravenous infusion in congestive heart failure and cardiac arrhythmia not responding to other drugs.

Glucophage. Metformin, *q.v.*

glucose. Dextrose, *q.v.*

glutethimide. Hypnotic of medium intensity and duration of action and a useful alternative to the barbiturates. Dose 1 to 2 tablets (250 to 500 mg) at night.

Glutril. Glibornuride, *q.v.*

glycerin, glycerol. A clear syrupy liquid used as a sweetening agent in mixtures and linctuses. It promotes drainage when applied to inflamed areas, and is used as a paste with magnesium sulphate for boils. It is frequently used in the form of suppositories for constipation.

glyceryl trinitrate. A vasodilator used mainly in angina pectoris as tablets 0·5 mg, which should be dissolved under the tongue for rapid absorption and prompt effect. A long-acting form is available as Sustac. Tolerance may occur with prolonged use, and the drug should be used with care in coronary thrombosis.

glycyrrhiza (liquorice). Used as an expectorant in cough mixtures, and to cover taste of nauseous drugs. Also has some anti-inflammatory properties (carbenoxolone, *q.v.*).

glymidine. An oral hypoglycaemic agent, chemically unrelated to tolbutamide, but with a similar action in mild, late-onset diabetes. Initial dose 3 g, maintenance dose 0·5 to 1·5 g. It may be used with other hypoglycaemic agents.

Gondafon. Glymidine, *q.v.*

gramicidin. A mixture of antibiotics effective against many Gram-positive organisms, but it is too toxic for systemic use. Used topically in infected skin conditions, often in association with neomycin and hydrocortisone.

griseofulvin. An orally active antifungal antibiotic. It is deposited selectively in the skin, hair and nails, and prevents further fungal invasion. Widely used in ringworm and tinea infections, but prolonged treatment is necessary. May cause headache, allergic reactions and gastric disturbance. Dose 0·5 to 1 g daily.

Grisovin. Griseofulvin, *q.v.*

guanethidine. A valuable antihypertensive drug with a powerful and prolonged action. It brings about a smooth reduction in bloodpressure by blocking transmission in adrenergic nerves, and it is widely employed in the treatment of all types of hypertension, often with a thiazide diuretic. Dose 10 mg daily, increased by 10 mg at weekly intervals according to response, with average doses of 50 to 75 mg daily, although sometimes much larger doses are required. Diarrhoea, weakness and bradycardia are common side-effects. Guanethidine is occasionally used as eye-drops in glaucoma and thyrotoxicosis.

guanoclor. An antihypertensive drug that may be effective in patients not responding adequately to other drugs. Dose 5 mg twice a day, increased as necessary up to 40 mg daily. Occasionally much larger doses may be required.

guanoxan. An antihypertensive drug similar in action to guanethidine, *q.v.* Useful in hypertension not responding to other drugs, but may cause liver damage. Dose 10 to 50 mg daily.

H

halibut-liver oil. A rich source of vitamins A and D. Dose 0·2 to 0·5 ml.

haloperidol. A tranquillizer chemically unrelated to chlorpromazine, but having a basically similar action. Valuable in mania and schizophrenic excitement. Dose 3 to 9 mg or more daily.

halothane. An inhalation anaesthetic more powerful than chloroform or ether, and largely free from the disadvantages of those older drugs. Not inflammable or explosive. Should not be used in pregnancy, or for patients with cardiac irregularities or liver damage.

Hartmann's solution. An electrolyte replacement solution containing sodium lactate, sodium chloride, potassium chloride, and calcium chloride; given orally or intravenously in acidosis and gastroenteritis.

helium. An inert gas. Occasionally used with oxygen in status asthmaticus.

Heminevrin. Chlormethiazole, *q.v.*

heparin. The natural anticoagulant obtained from lung and liver tissue. It is widely used in the treatment of postoperative thrombosis and thromboembolic diseases. It is given by intravenous injec-tion and the action is prompt but brief, so four-hourly injections are necessary to maintain the effect. Toxic reactions are few and slight. Dose 5,000 to 15,000 units. Intramuscular injections are painful and less reliable. Overdosage can be controlled by the intravenous injection of protamine sulphate, *q.v.* Treatment with heparin may be combined with that of oral anticoagulants such as ethyl biscoumacetate, *q.v.*, phenindione, *q.v.*, or warfarin, *q.v.*, to provide immediate action before the slow-acting oral drugs begin to take effect.

heroin. Diamorphine, *q.v.*

Herpid. Idoxuridine, *q.v.*

hexachlorophene. An antiseptic used for skin sterilization, and present in some medicated soaps. Its safety has been questioned, especially when used as a dusting powder for babies.

hexamine. A formaldehyde derivative of low toxicity used as a urinary antiseptic. Now largely replaced by the sulphonamides, but is of value when more potent drugs are contraindicated. Dose 0·6 to 2 g. Usually given in association with mandelic acid, *q.v.*, or as Hiprex, *q.v.*

hexoestrol. A synthetic oestrogen similar to stilboestrol, *q.v.*, but less active. Dose 1 to 5 mg.

Hexopal. Inositol nicotinate, *q.v.*

hexylresorcinol. A useful vermifuge of low toxicity for expelling roundworms, hookworms, threadworms and flukes. Adult anthelmintic dose 1 g, given on an empty stomach, followed by a saline purge. Piperazine, *q.v.*, is now preferred for the removal of threadworm and roundworm.

Hibitane. Chlorhexidine, *q.v.*

Hiprex. A compound of hexamine and hippuric acid that provides adequate acidification of the urine and consequent antibacterial action. Of value in chronic urinary infections, and for prophylaxis before and after urological surgery.

histamine. A compound present in a bound form in all mammalian tissues; its release is probably the ultimate cause of many allergic conditions. It has been used in circulatory disorders and as it stimulates gastric secretion, it is given to detect achlorhydria. Dose 0·5 to 1 mg by subcutaneous or intramuscular injection. In gastric function tests larger doses are sometimes given in association with an antihistamine which reduces the systemic effects of histamine without influencing the effects on gastric secretion.

Histantin. Chlorcyclizine, *q.v.*

homatropine. An atropine derivative with a similar but more rapid mydriatic action (15 to 30 minutes), but a shorter duration of effect. Solution (2%) is often used with cocaine, which increases the effect.

Honvan. Fosfesterol, *q.v.*

Hyalase. Hyaluronidase, *q.v.*

hyaluronidase. A 'spreading' factor derived from testes. When intravenous drip infusion of an electrolyte solution is impracticable, the injection of 1 mg of hyaluronidase will promote the absorption of 500 to 1,000 ml of electrolyte solution by subcutaneous drip infusion.

hydrallazine. A synthetic drug with useful antihypertensive properties. It is given in essential and malignant hypertension, usually in association with a thiazide diuretic, and is also of value in the toxaemia of pregnancy. Dose 12·5 mg initially, four times a day, slowly increased to 100 mg as required. Also given by intravenous drip in doses of 20 to 40 mg in emergency such as preeclampsia.

Hydrenox. Hydroflumethiazide, *q.v.*

hydrochlorothiazide. One of the most useful of the thiazide diuretics. It brings about a marked increase in the excretion of salts and water, and is of considerable value in congestive heart failure, and other oedematous conditions. The drug also increases the excretion of potassium as well as sodium, and if treatment is prolonged, some potassium replacement therapy will be necessary, either as potassium chloride, *q.v.*, or as effervescent potassium tablets. Hydrochlorothiazide is also useful in hypertension as it potentiates the action of other drugs. Dose 25 to 50 mg.

hydrocortisone. A derivative of cortisone, *q.v.*, with marked anti-inflammatory effects, particularly when applied locally. Widely employed in inflammatory skin, eye and ear conditions, sometimes in association with antibiotics such as neomycin, to reduce secondary bacterial invasion. Ointments should be applied thinly in strengths from 0·5 to 1%. Frequently given by intra-articular injection in bursitis and associated conditions. Of great value in status asthmaticus, allergic emergencies and shock-like states when given intravenously in doses of 100 mg.

hydroflumethiazide. A diuretic similar in action and uses to hydrochlorothiazide, *q.v.* Dose 25 to 100 mg.

hydrogen peroxide solution. Contains 5 to 7% H_2O_2, giving about 20 volumes of oxygen. A deodorizing antiseptic used mainly for cleaning wounds. Also used as a mouthwash (diluted 1 to 7) and ear-drops (1 in 4 in water or 50% alcohol).

HydroSaluric. Hydrochlorothiazide, *q.v.*

hydrous wool fat. Wool fat containing 30% of water. Also known as lanolin. It is used as a constituent of water-in-oil ointment bases and related emollient products.

hydroxocobalamin. A drug closely related to cyanocobalamin, *q.v.*, but is excreted much more slowly. Adequate blood levels in pernicious and megaloblastic anaemia can be maintained by a monthly injection of 250 micrograms.

Hygroton. Chlorthalidone, *q.v.*

hyoscine. Also known as scopolamine. An alkaloid obtained from plants of the belladonna group. It is a powerful hypnotic and is widely used together with papaveretum for pre-medication before operation. Also has anti-emetic properties, and is useful in travel sickness. Dose 0·3 to 0·6 mg.

hyoscine butylbromide. A derivative of hyoscine that resembles atropine in its antispasmodic action, but differs in lacking any action on the central nervous system. Useful in spasm and hypermotility of the gastro-intestinal tract. Dose 10 to 20 mg.

hyoscyamus. The dried leaves of henbane. It has actions similar to those of belladonna, and is used mainly with saline diuretics such as potassium citrate to relieve spasm. Dose of tincture, 2 to 4 ml.

Hypovase. Prazosin, *q.v.*

I

ibuprofen. An anti-inflammatory and analgesic agent widely used in the treatment of rheumatoid arthritis and similar conditions. Is generally well tolerated, but care is necessary in peptic ulcer, liver dysfunction and asthma. Dose 1200 mg daily initially, adjusted to maintenance doses of 600 mg or more.

ichthammol. A thick, dark brown liquid with a characteristic odour, derived from certain bituminous oils. It is a mild antiseptic and is used in ointments, and as solution (10%) in glycerin for ulcers and inflamed areas.

ichthyol. Ichthammol, *q.v.*

idoxuridine. An antiviral agent used locally in dendritic ulcers of the eye as drops of 0·1% solution or 0·5% ointment. Has also been used intravenously for systemic viral infections.

Ilotycin. Erythromycin, *q.v.*

Imferon. An iron-dextran preparation for intramuscular injection. Used in iron-deficiency anaemias when oral iron preparations are not tolerated. Dose 5 ml daily, or on alternate days, according to degree of haemoglobin deficiency. The total amount so required is occasionally given as a single dose by slow intravenous drip infusion, but reactions have followed such total dose infusions.

imipramine. A tricyclic psychotherapeutic drug with powerful and specific antidepressant properties. Response to the drug may be slow, and long treatment is often necessary. Dose 25 mg three times a day, gradually increased to 50 mg as required. Imipramine should not be given in association with or soon after monoamine oxidase inhibitors, as the effects of both drugs may be increased.

Imodium. Loperamide, *q.v.*

Imuran. Azathioprine, *q.v.*

Inderal. Propranolol, *q.v.*

indigo carmine. A blue dye used as a 0·4% solution by injection as a renal function test. Normally the urine is coloured blue in ten minutes or so.

Indocid. Indomethacin, *q.v.*

indomethacin. An anti-inflammatory and analgesic drug of value in many arthritic and rheumatoid conditions, and in acute gout. It may cause gastro-intestinal disturbance. Administration as suppository gives a prolonged action, and is useful at night to reduce morning stiffness. Dose 25 to 50 mg orally, 100 mg as suppository.

inositol nicotinate. A peripheral vasodilator similar to tolazoline, q.v. Dose 400 mg to 1 g.

insulin. The antidiabetic principle of the pancreas, regulating the metabolism of carbohydrates and fats. It is widely used by subcutaneous injection in the treatment of diabetes mellitus. A number of varieties of insulin are available, designed to extend the action of the drug, reduce the frequency of injections, and so simulate the effects of the natural hormone more closely. These include protamine-zinc-insulin, globin-insulin, and insulin-zinc-suspensions ('Lente insulins'). The latter are free from added protein and so less likely to cause local reactions. Dosage is based entirely on the patients requirements. In diabetic emergency, soluble insulin remains the preparation of choice.

Intal. Sodium cromoglycate, q.v.

Integrin. Oxypertine, q.v.

Intralipid. An emulsion of soya oil, specially prepared for slow intravenous injection when a high-calorie intake is required, as in severe malnutrition.

Intraval Sodium. Thiopentone sodium, q.v.

Inversine. Mecamylamine, q.v.

iodine. Powerful antiseptic used as tincture of iodine for skin preparation. Given orally as Lugol's solution, q.v., in pre-operative treatment of thyrotoxicosis. Dose: as Aqueous Iodine Solution (Lugol's Solution) 0·1 to 1 ml; as Weak Iodine Solution (tincture of iodine) 0·6 to 2 ml.

iodized oil. Poppy-seed oil containing 40% iodine in combination. Used as contrast agent in X-ray examination of bronchial tract, uterus, fistulae, etc. The oil decomposes and darkens slowly on storage, and only colourless or pale yellow material should be used.

iodoform. Yellow powder with strong odour. Mild antiseptic, used mainly as B.I.P.P., q.v., for application to abscesses and ulcers.

iopanoic acid. A radio-opaque substance used as a contrast agent in cholecystography. It is largely excreted in the bile when given orally. Dose 2 to 6 g.

ipecacuanha. The dried root

from which emetine, q.v., is obtained. It has expectorant and emetic properties, and is used mainly as the tincture (ipecacuanha wine). Dose 0·25 to 1 ml; emetic dose, 5 to 20 ml.

iron and ammonium citrate. A water-soluble iron complex with little astringent or gastric irritant effect. Now largely replaced by tablet preparations of iron. Dose 1 to 3 g.

iron gluconate. Ferrous gluconate. One of the most widely used preparations for iron-deficiency anaemias. It is less irritating than ferrous sulphate and is a useful alternative when the sulphate is not tolerated. Prophylactic dose 600 mg daily; therapeutic dose 2·4 to 4·8 g daily.

iron sulphate. Ferrous sulphate. Used extensively in iron-deficiency anaemias as it is effective in small doses, and fairly well tolerated but may cause gastric disturbance in some patients. Usually given as tablets, each containing 200 mg. These tablets are potentially dangerous for small children as death has occurred after accidental administration.

Ismelin. Guanethidine, q.v.

isocarboxazid. A monoamine oxidase inhibitor used in the treatment of exogenous and reactive depression. Long treatment may be necessary to achieve full remission of symptoms. Dose 10 to 30 mg daily.

isoetharine. A bronchodilator similar to isoprenaline, q.v., but with a longer action. Dose 10 to 30 mg daily.

I-so-gel. Red granules of mucilage from various seeds, for use as a bulk-increasing laxative. Dose 2 to 4 g or more.

isoniazid. A pyridine derivative with a specific action against Mycobacterium tuberculosis. Widely used in the treatment of pulmonary and other forms of tuberculosis, but as bacterial resistance soon develops, combined treatment with other antitubercular drugs is essential. Side-effects include nausea and peripheral neuritis. Dose 300 to 600 mg daily.

isoprenaline sulphate. A compound related to adrenaline, but with increased bronchodilator and reduced vasoconstrictor potency. Widely used in asthma, bronchospasm, etc., by oral inhalation from special aerosol inhalers, or as sublingual tablets (20 mg). Side-effects include tachycardia and nausea.

isopropyl alcohol. Colourless inflammable liquid. Has been used as a pre-operative antiseptic.

Isoxyl. Thiocarlide, q.v.

Izal. An antiseptic emulsion of tar-oils. Diluted 1:600 for use as a general purpose bactericide.

J

Jectofer. A soluble complex of iron, sorbitol, citric acid and dextrin. Used by intramuscular injection in iron-deficiency anaemias in doses of 2 ml daily, the total dose being based on the degree of haemoglobin deficiency.

K

kanamycin. An antibiotic related to neomycin, but less toxic and so suitable for systemic use. It is given by intramuscular injection in severe infections due to Gram-negative and Gram-positive organisms particularly those resistant to other antibiotics. Dose 1 to 2 g daily in divided doses. Dose must be carefully adjusted to avoid neurotoxic reactions and possible deafness.

Kannasyn. Kanamycin, q.v.

Kantrex. Kanamycin, q.v.

kaolin. Native aluminium silicate. Used as an adsorbent in diarrhoea, colitis, food poisoning, etc., and as a dusting powder Dose 15 to 50 g.

Keflex. Cephalexin, q.v.

Kefzol. Cephazolin, q.v.

Keflin. Cephalothin, q.v.

Kelfizine. Sulfametopyrazine, q.v.

Kemadrin. Procyclidine, q.v.

Kenalog. Triamcinolone, q.v.

Kerecid. Idoxuridine, q.v.

Ketalar. Ketamine, q.v.

ketamine. A short-acting intravenous anaesthetic with analgesic properties. It is given in doses of 2 mg per kg body-weight, and produces anaesthesia in about 30 seconds, which lasts 5 to 10 minutes. Anaesthesia can be maintained if necessary by other anaesthetic drugs. The analgesic action of ketamine is useful in certain neurodiagnostic procedures, and in the treatment of severe burns. Care should be taken not to disturb the patient during the post-anaesthetic period, as vivid dreams or hallucinations may occur during the recovery phase.

ketoprofen. An anti-inflammatory and analgesic agent used in rheumatoid arthritis, gout, spondylitis and related conditions. Generally well tolerated, but should be given with food. Care is necessary in peptic ulcer and hepatic disease. May increase the action of anticoagulants and other drugs bound to plasma protein. Like aspirin, it is an inhibitor of prostaglandin synthesis. Dose 100 to 200 mg daily.

Konakion. Vitamin K$_1$, q.v.

L

lachesine. An atropine substitute with mydriatic properties. Used mainly as a 1% solution in cases of atropine irritation.

lactoflavin. Riboflavine, q.v.

lactose. The sugar present in milk. It is less soluble and less sweet than ordinary sugar. It is widely used in tablet making as a diluent and excipient.

lactulose. A sugar that is not absorbed by the gastrointestinal tract. Used in the treatment of chronic constipation and hepatic encephalopathy. Dose 5 to 20 g daily.

laevulose (fructose). An easily digested sugar, particularly for diabetics as it can be converted to glycogen in the absence of insulin. Sometimes given intravenously as an alternative to dextrose.

Lamprene. Clofazimine, q.v.

lanatoside. C. A cardiac glycoside from *Digitalis lanata*. It is excreted more rapidly than some digitalis products and so has a wider margin of safety. Dose 1 to 1·5 mg orally, for rapid digitalization, followed by maintenance doses of 0·25 to 0·75 mg daily.

Lanette wax. A mixture of cetyl and stearyl alcohols with emulsifying properties. It is added to soft paraffin ointment bases to produce water-miscible products.

lanolin. Hydrous wool fat, q.v.

Lanoxin. Digoxin, q.v.

Lanvis. Thioguanine, q.v.

Largactil. Chlorpromazine, q.v.

Larodopa. Levodopa, q.v.

Lasix. Frusemide, q.v.

Lassar's paste. A stiff ointment containing zinc oxide, starch and white soft paraffin with 2% salicylic acid. Used as protective in eczema.

laudanum. Tincture of opium; contains morphine 1%. Dose 0·3 to 2 ml.

Ledercort. Triamcinolone, q.v.

Lederkyn. Sulphamethoxypyridazine, q.v.

Ledermycin. A tetracycline derivative with the wide range of activity of the parent compound, but more active. Dose 150 mg six-hourly.

Lentizol. Amitriptyline, q.v.

leptazol. A respiratory and cardiac stimulant; has been used in respiratory failure during anaesthesia. Dose 100 mg by injection.

Lethidrone. Nalorphine, q.v.

Leukeran. Chlorambucil, q.v.

levallorphan. A morphine antagonist which in small doses is claimed to inhibit the respiratory depression induced by morphine and related drugs. Used in combination with pethidine in obstetrics to reduce anoxia of the newborn.

levodopa. An amino-acid that is converted to dopamine in the body. It is used in the treatment of Parkinson's disease, which is associated with a reduction in brain dopamine levels. Side-effects include nausea, dizziness and psychiatric disturbance. Dose 0·5 g daily initially, slowly increasing according to response to 6 to 9 g daily.

Levophed. Solution of noradrenaline, q.v., for treatment of shock. Given by slow intravenous injection after 1:250 dilution with saline.

levorphanol. Powerful analgesic similar to morphine, effective both orally and by injection. Tablets of 1·5 mg, ampoules of 2 mg, for intramuscular or subcutaneous injection.

Librium. Chlordiazepoxide, q.v.

lignocaine. A local anaesthetic similar to procaine, but with a more intense and extended effect. Used for infiltration anaesthesia as 0·5 to 2% solution, usually with adrenaline. Widely used in dentistry. A 2 to 4% solution is used for local application before bronchoscopy.

Lincocin. Lincomycin, q.v.

lincomycin. An orally active antibiotic with a range of activity similar to that of erythromycin. Well absorbed and widely distributed in tissues, bone and pleural fluids, and excreted in urine. Dose 500 mg four times a day before meals; in severe conditions 600 mg or more twice daily by intramuscular or intravenous injection.

Lioresal. Baclofen, q.v.

liothyronine. A hormone of the thyroid gland, and probably the substance into which thyroxine, q.v., is converted. Useful in patients not responding to thyroxine. Dose 5 to 100 micrograms daily.

Lipiodol. Iodized oil, q.v.

lithium carbonate. Used in the prophylaxis of manic-depressive disease. The mode of action is not known. Dose 0·25 to 1·5 g daily.

liquorice. Glycyrrhiza, q.v.

Lomodex. Dextran, q.v.

loperamide. A synthetic inhibitor of peristalsis, of value in the treatment of acute diarrhoea. Dose 4 mg initially, followed by three or four doses of 2 mg to a maximum daily dose of 16 mg.

Lopresor. Metoprolol, q.v.

lorazepam. An antidepressant useful in anxiety and tension states not responding to other drugs. Dose 1 to 10 mg daily.

Lorfan. Levallorphan, q.v.

Lucidril. Meclofenoxate, q.v.

Lugol's solution. An aqueous

solution of iodine 5%, potassium iodide 10%. Used in the pre-operative treatment of thyrotoxicosis. Dose 0·3 to 1 ml.

Luminal. Phenobarbitone, *q.v.*

Lynoral. Ethinyloestradiol, *q.v.*

Lysivaine. Ethopropazine, *q.v.*

lysol. A solution of cresol, *q.v.*, 50% in a liquid soap. It is a powerful but caustic disinfectant, but care must be taken that it does not come in contact with the skin. Related but less caustic preparations are represented by Sudol and Printol.

M

Macrodex. Dextran, *q.v.*

Madribon. Sulphadimethoxine, *q.v.*

Magmilor. Nifuratel, *q.v.*

magnesium carbonate. A white, insoluble powder with antacid and laxative properties. Dose 0·6 to 4 g.

magnesium hydroxide. A mild antacid laxative, usually given in aqueous suspension as Cream of Magnesia, although tablet forms are also available. It is often preferred to magnesium carbonate, as no release of carbon dioxide and consequent gastric distension follows its use. Cream of Magnesia is a useful antidote in mineral acid poisoning.

magnesium sulphate (Epsom salts). A powerful saline aperient, producing loose stools by preventing the reabsorption of water. Used externally for the treatment of boils and carbuncles as a paste with glycerin.

magnesium trisilicate. A white insoluble powder, with mild but prolonged antacid effects. It is widely employed for the treatment of peptic ulcer, often in association with other antacids. Dose 0·3 to 2 g.

Mandelamine. Hexamine mandelate, referred to under mandelic acid, *q.v.*

mandelic acid. Used as ammonium or hexamine mandelate as a bacteriostat in *E. coli* infections of the urinary tract when more powerful drugs are not tolerated. The urine must be kept acid, and the additional use of ammonium chloride or sodium acid phosphate may be required. Dose 2 to 4 g.

Mandl's paint. A solution of iodine in glycerin. Used occasionally in tonsillitis as an antiseptic throat paint.

Mandrax. Methaqualone, *q.v.*, and diphenhydramine, used in insomnia. Available as tablets or capsules.

mannitol hexanitrate. A vasodilator of mild but prolonged action similar to erythrityl tetranitrate, *q.v.* Dose 15 to 60 mg.

mannomustine. A combination of mustine, *q.v.*, with the sugar mannitol. Such combination reduces the severe irritant effects of mustine, and the product, although usually given by intravenous injection, is occasionally used orally. Dose 100 mg.

Marboran. Methisazone, *q.v.*

Marcain. Bupivacaine, *q.v.*

Marevan. Warfarin, *q.v.*

Marplan. Isocarboxazid, *q.v.*

Masteril. Drostanolone, *q.v.*

Maxolon. Metoclopramide, *q.v.*

mazindol. An appetite depressant for use in obesity. Care is necessary if used with antihypertensive drugs, and antidepressants of the monoamine oxidase inhibitor type. Dose 2 mg daily after breakfast.

mebhydrolin. An antihistamine used in hayfever, urticaria and other allergic conditions. Dose 50 to 100 mg three times a day.

mecamylamine. A ganglionic blocking agent used in the treatment of hypertension. Dose 2·5 mg twice daily, increased according to need and response to an average daily dose of 25 mg. Now largely replaced by drugs of the guanethidine type.

Mechothane. A derivative of carbachol, *q.v.*, and used for

similar purposes. Dose 30 to 120 mg daily.

meclofenoxate. A central stimulant, used in mental confusion, depression and melancholia, and in delirium tremens. Has also been used in anoxia and coma. Dose 300 mg four times a day.

medazepam. A tranquillizing agent similar to chlordiazepoxide, *q.v.* Used in anxiety and tension states, and in alcoholism. Dose 15 to 40 mg daily.

mefenamic acid. An analgesic drug with anti-inflammatory properties, useful in arthritis and rheumatoid conditions. May cause gastro-intestinal disturbance. Dose 250 mg four times a day.

mefruside. A diuretic with a slower and more prolonged action than related drugs. Useful in the long-term treatment of oedema, in hypertension and pre-menstrual tension. Dose 12·5 to 50 mg daily, according to need and response. A potassium supplement may be required. Care is necessary in renal and hepatic deficiency.

Megaclor. Clomocycline, *q.v.*

Megimide. Bemegride, *q.v.*

Melleril. Thioridazine, *q.v.*

melphalan. A cytostatic drug with an action similar to mustine, *q.v.* Used in multiple myeloma, and by isolated perfusion in malignant melanoma. Oral dose 10 to 30 mg; by perfusion 70 to 100 mg.

menaphthone. An oil-soluble synthetic vitamin K, q.v. Menaphthone is used in haemorrhage due to hypoprothrombinaemia, and in obstructive jaundice. Dose 1 to 10 mg daily by intramuscular injection.

menthol. Colourless crystals obtained from oil of peppermint. Used as spray or drops for naso-pharyngeal inflammation, and as an inhalation, often with friar's balsam, for the relief of coryza and catarrh.

mepacrine. A synthetic antimalarial, similar to quinine in its general effects. Now replaced by chloroquine, q.v., proguanil, q.v., and other powerful antimalarial drugs. Dose: prophylactic, 0·1 g daily; therapeutic, 0·2 to 0·5 g daily.

Mepavlon. Meprobamate, q.v.

mephenesin. A synthetic muscle relaxant, used in the treatment of spastic conditions and muscle spasm. Dose, orally, 0·5 to 1 g.

mepivacaine. A local anaesthetic similar to lignocaine, q.v. It has no vasodilator action, and may be used without the addition of adrenaline.

meprobamate. A mild tranquil-

lizing drug with muscle-relaxant properties. Indicated in neurotic and tension states, alcoholism and associated conditions. Dose 400 mg three to four times a day.

mepyramine maleate. One of the less potent antihistamines, and with a shorter action than promethazine, q.v. It is used in the treatment of allergic conditions such as urticaria, hay-fever, drug reactions and itching skin conditions. It may cause sensitization, and topical use is now less popular. It is given by injection in severe allergic conditions, and in the 'augmented histamine test' for gastric function. Dose 100 to 200 mg.

Merbentyl. Dicyclomine, q.v.

mercaptopurine. A cytotoxic agent used in the treatment of acute leukaemia and chronic myelogenous leukaemia. The best results are obtained in children. Close haematological control throughout treatment is essential. Dose 2·5 mg per kg bodyweight daily.

mercuric oxide. A bright yellow powder with antiseptic properties. Once used as golden eye ointment, for the treatment of conjunctivitis and blepharitis.

mercurochrome. A red dye with

weak antiseptic properties. Used occasionally for skin sterilization.

mersalyl. A powerful mercurial diuretic, once used extensively in oedema due to cardiac failure, but now largely replaced by the thiazide diuretics. Dose 0·5 to 2 ml by deep intramuscular injection repeated after three or four days.

Merthiolate. Thiomersal, *q.v.*

Mesontoin. Methoin, *q.v.*

Mestinon. Pyridostigmine, *q.v.*

metaraminol. A vasopressor drug with a powerful and prolonged action. Of great value in the hypotension of shock, haemorrhage, myocardial infarction and infection. Is suitable for intramuscular or subcutaneous injection as unlike noradrenaline it does not cause local tissue damage. May also be given by slow intravenous drip infusion after dilution with saline or dextrose solution. Dose 2 to 10 mg.

metformin. An orally active hypoglycaemic agent similar in action to phenformin, *q.v.* Dose 1·5 g daily, adjusted according to need and response.

methacholine. A derivative of acetylcholine, used in peripheral vascular disorders, and for paroxysmal auricular tachycardia. Dose 100 to 200 mg orally; 10 to 25 mg by subcutaneous injection.

methacycline. A tetracycline derivative with the general antibacterial action of that group of drugs. Dose 150 mg.

methadone. A synthetic analgesic resembling morphine in its general effects, but its sedative action is less marked. It is also a cough-centre depressant, and is of value in the treatment of severe and useless cough. Dose 5 to 10 mg orally, or by subcutaneous or intramuscular injection.

methandienone. A non-virilizing androgen, used in osteoporosis and protein deficiency states. Dose 5 to 10 mg.

methaqualone. A sedative and hypnotic drug given for insomnia as an alternative to the barbiturates. Dose 75 to 300 mg.

methicillin. A penicillin derivative not destroyed by the enzyme penicillinase, and so effective against otherwise resistant staphylococci. Less effective than benzyl penicillin against penicillin-sensitive streptococci. The drug is not effective orally, and is usually given by intramuscular injection in doses of 1 g four to six-hourly. May be given intravenously in severe infections. Cloxacillin, *q.v.*, and flucloxacillin, *q.v.*, are related drugs effective orally.

methionine. A sulphur-containing amino-acid essential for nutrition. It is sometimes used in toxic hepatitis and to increase the effects of urinary antiseptics by increasing the acidity of the urine. Dose 3 to 10 g daily.

methisazone. An antiviral drug that appears to inhibit the synthesis of viral protein. Used mainly in the prophylaxis of those who have been in contact with smallpox patients. Useful for mass prophylaxis. Dose 3 g twice a day for one day.

methixene. A drug used in the treatment of parkinsonism, but relieves the tremor more than the rigidity. It may be given with other drugs to evoke a full response. Dose 15 to 60 mg daily.

methohexitone. An intravenous anaesthetic similar to thiopentone, *q.v.*, but with a very short action and quick recovery rate. Used for induction anaesthesia or minor operations. Dose 50 to 120 mg.

methoin. An anticonvulsant similar to phenytoin, used mainly in the treatment of grand mal. Side-effects such as drowsiness are more frequent than with phenytoin, and blood changes may also occur. Dose 50 to 100 mg.

methotrexate. A folic acid antagonist used in the treatment of leukaemia, breast cancer and other cancerous states. May be given orally, as a daily dose of 2·5 to 5 mg, or a weekly dose of 25 mg. May also be given by intramuscular injection.

methoxamine. A blood-pressure-raising compound used in the hypotension following spinal anaesthesia and post-operative shock. It has little cardiac or central stimulant action. Dose 10 to 15 mg by intravenous or intramuscular injection.

methsuximide. An anticonvulsant used mainly in petit mal and psychomotor epilepsy, often with other drugs. Of no value in grand mal. Dose 300 mg daily, later adjusted to a maximum of 1·2 g daily.

methyclothiazide. A diuretic similar to chlorothiazide, but with increased potency. Dose 2·5 to 10 mg daily.

methyl cellulose. A derivative of cellulose that forms stable, mucilaginous solutions in water. Used as emulsifying agent, jelly base and bulk laxative.

methylamphetamine. A central stimulant similar to amphetamine sulphate, occasionally used as a pressor agent in spinal anaesthesia, and in poisoning by barbiturates.

Dose 10 to 30 mg by intramuscular or intravenous injection.

methylated spirit. Alcohol containing 5% of wood naphtha. Used for skin preparation and alcoholic applications. The methylated spirit used domestically is less pure, and is coloured violet to indicate its unsuitability for medicinal use.

methyldopa. A potent hypotensive compound used in the treatment of hypertensive cardiovascular conditions. The drug produces a smooth reduction in blood-pressure that is not significantly affected by exercise. The action is increased by the administration of thiazide diuretics. Drowsiness may occur during the early stages of treatment. Dose 0·5 to 2 g daily.

methylpentynol. A short-acting hypnotic. It has some antiapprehensive properties, and is useful in emotional stress. Dose 0·25 to 1 g.

methyl phenidate. A central stimulant less powerful than the amphetamines, useful in narcolepsy and some psychiatric conditions. Dose 10 mg.

methyl salicylate. Pale yellow liquid with characteristic odour. It has the analgesic properties of the salicylates, but is too toxic for systemic use, and is used solely for external application as liniment or ointment.

methyltestosterone. An orally active form of testosterone. Tablets should be dissolved under the tongue for maximum absorption. Dose 5 to 50 mg daily in divided doses.

methyprylone. A synthetic sedative and hypnotic with actions and uses similar to those of chloral, q.v. Dose 200 to 400 mg.

methysergide. A synthetic drug related to ergometrine, but used empirically in the prophylaxis of migraine. Of no value in an acute attack. Dose 2 to 6 mg daily.

metoclopramide. An anti-emetic of value in drug-induced nausea and vomiting. Of little use in travel sickness. Also used to induce gastric peristalsis during X-ray examination of the stomach. Dose 5 to 10 mg.

metoprolol. A beta-blocking agent, q.v., mainly used in the control of angina, but also of value in hypertension. Dose in angina 50 to 100 mg thrice daily, in hypertension doses up to 200 mg twice daily may be required. Care is necessary in heart block, bradycardia and pulmonary disease.

metronidazole. An orally effective drug for the treatment of

vaginal and urethral tricho-
moniasis. Dose 200 mg three
times a day for seven days.
Also used in acute intestinal
amoebiasis in daily doses of
2·4 g for two days.

mexiletine. An antiarrhythmic
drug that depresses excessive
myocardial activity with little
action on normal function.
Used in the prophylaxis and
control of ventricular arrhythmia. Initial dose 400 to 600
mg, with maintenance doses
of 200 to 250 mg. Also given
by intravenous infusion in
doses of 200 to 250 mg.

Mexitil. Mexiletine, *q.v.*

mianserin. An antidepressant
with reduced anticholinergic
side-effects. Useful in all types
of depression, including
those where anxiety is also
present. It should not be used
with monoamine oxidase inhibitors, *q.v.*, or barbiturates.
In epileptics, the dose of anticonvulsant may have to be
increased. Dose 10 mg twice
a day, increased as needed to
30 to 60 mg daily

Midamor. Amiloride, *q.v.*

Midicel. Sulphamethoxypyridazine, *q.v.*

Milontin. Phensuximide, *q.v.*

Milton. A stable solution of
sodium hypochlorite with
sodium chloride. Dilutions of
2·5 to 5% form antiseptic
solutions of considerable use-
fulness.

Miltown. Meprobamate, *q.v.*

Minocin. Minocycline, *q.v.*

minocycline. A tetracycline derivative with the wide range
of activity of the tetracycline
antibiotics, but with a longer
action. Dose 200 mg initially,
followed by 100 mg twice
daily.

Minodiab. Glipizide, *q.v.*

Mintezol. Thiabendazole, *q.v.*

Modecate. Fluphenazine, *q.v.*

Moditen. Fluphenazine, *q.v.*

Mogadon. Nitrazepam, *q.v.*

**monoamine oxidase inhibitors
(M.A.O.I.).** Monoamine oxidase is an enzyme concerned
with the breakdown of serotonin, noradrenaline and
adrenaline. Chemically, these
substances are amines, and
they are stored in many organs
of the body, including the
brain, where they are liber-
ated as required to function
as transmitters of nerve impulses. The period for which
they act is short, as they are
rapidly broken down to
simpler substances by monoamine oxidase. An inhibition
of the enzyme would permit
an increase in the amount of
these amines in the brain,
and such an increase is associated with cerebral stimulation. On that basis, several
enzyme inhibitors have been
used in the treatment of
depression, although the
mode of action is probably far

more complex than the simple one indicated above. These inhibitors have an extensive pharmacological action, and can increase the effects of pressor drugs, analgesics, anaesthetics, sedatives, C.N.S. stimulants, and many other drugs. Even certain foods, particularly cheese, may cause a dangerous rise in blood-pressure during M.A.O.I. therapy. Great care is necessary during combined therapy, and ideally 10 to 14 days should elapse after ceasing M.A.O.I. treatment before using other potent drugs. Examples of monoamine oxidase inhibitors are iproniazid (Marsilid), isocarboxazid (Marplan), nialamide (Niamid), phenelzine (Nardil) and tranylcypromine (Parnate).

morphine. The principal alkaloid of opium. It is widely used for severe pain and the associated anxiety and stress, and in cardiac asthma, shock and blood loss. It also checks cough and reduces peristalsis, but may cause nausea and vomiting. Morphine is more active by injection than orally. It may increase an established respiratory depression, and that condition is a contra-indication. Tolerance of the drug, and dangers of dependence, should be borne in mind if treatment is prolonged. Dose 8 to 20 mg.

Motival. Fluphenazine, *q.v.*

mustine. An organic compound with cytostatic effects on growing cells similar to those produced by X-rays. It is used in Hodgkin's disease and other neoplastic conditions. Solutions, which must be freshly prepared, are given by slow intravenous drip. Injection outside a vein causes very severe inflammation. Occasionally given by intrapleural injection in bronchial carcinoma. Average dose 5 to 8 mg.

Myambutol. Ethambutol, *q.v.*

Myanesin. Mephenesin, *q.v.*

Mycivin. Lincomycin, *q.v.*

Myleran. Busulphan, *q.v.*

Myocrisin. Sodium aurothiomalate, *q.v.*

Myodil. An oily iodine compound used in myelography. Injected intrathecally in doses of 2 to 5 ml.

Mysoline. Primidone, *q.v.*

N

Nacton. Poldine, *q.v.*

nalidixic acid. A synthetic antibacterial drug. Following oral administration, the blood-levels are too low to be useful in systemic infections, but the drug is correspondingly of great value in urinary infections, especially those due to Gram-negative organisms. Dose 1 g six-hourly.

nalorphine. A specific antidote against the action of morphine, pethidine and associated drugs, and is useful in the treatment of overdose or unusual susceptibility. Respiration and blood-pressure are dramatically improved after intramuscular or intravenous injection. Dose 10 to 40 mg. Neonatal dose 0·25 to 1 mg.

naloxone. A more powerful antagonist of narcotic depression than nalorphine. Useful in the respiratory depression caused by narcotics, and in the diagnosis of acute narcotic poisoning. Dose 0·4 mg by intravenous or intramuscular injection. Children's doses 1·5 to 3 micrograms per kg or more according to age and need, repeated as required.

nandrolone. A steroid derivative, related to testosterone, but with markedly reduced virilizing properties. It has the anabolic or tissue-building properties of the parent compound, and is used in postoperative convalescence in both sexes. Also useful in osteoporosis and wasting diseases. Dose 25 mg weekly by intramuscular injection.

naphazoline hydrochloride. A vasoconstrictor used for the relief of inflammatory or allergic nasal congestion. It is used as a spray or drops (1:1,000) not more than four times a day.

Naprosyn. Naproxen, *q.v.*

naproxen. A non-steroidal anti-inflammatory agent useful as an alternative to other drugs in rheumatoid and similar conditions. Care is necessary in peptic ulcer. Dose 250 mg twice a day.

Narcan. Naloxone, *q.v.*

Nardil. Phenelzine. *See* monoamine oxidase inhibitors.

Narphen. Phenazocine, *q.v.*

Natulan. Procarbazine, *q.v.*

Navane. Thiothixene, *q.v.*

Navidrex. Cyclopenthiazide, *q.v.* Navidrex-K contains potassium chloride in addition, to offset any potassium loss in the urine caused by the diuretic action of cyclopenthiazide.

Nebcin. Tobramycin, *q.v.*

Negram. Nalidixic acid, *q.v.*

Nembutal. Pentobarbitone sodium, *q.v.*

Neo-Cytamen. Hydroxocobalamin, *q.v.*

Neo-mercazole. Carbimazole, *q.v.*

neomycin. An antibiotic active against a wide range of organisms, but owing to its toxic nature when injected, it is used mainly in preparations for external use. It is often combined with hydrocortisone in the treatment of in-flamed and infected areas. Occasionally used as an intestinal antiseptic. Dose 2 to 8 g daily in divided doses.

Neophryn. Phenylephrine, *q.v.*

neostigmine. An inhibitor of cholinesterase which thus indirectly prolongs the action of acetylcholine released at nerve endings. Valuable in the treatment of myasthenia gravis in doses of 15 to 30 mg. Widely used post-operatively to antagonize the residual effects of muscle relaxants of the tubocurarine and gallamine type in doses of 2·5 to 5 mg intravenously, after a preliminary injection of 0·5 to 1 mg of atropine.

Nepenthe. A proprietary preparation similar to tincture of opium.

Neptal. A mercurial diuretic similar in action to mersalyl, *q.v.*

Neulactil. Pericyazine, *q.v.*

nialamide. A monoamine oxidase inhibitor used in exogenous and reactive depression. If an initial response has been obtained within three to four weeks treatment should be prolonged to obtain a full remission. Dose 150 mg daily initially, reduced later to 75 mg.

Niamid. Nialamide, *q.v.*

niclosamide. A synthetic anthelmintic of value in the elimina-tion of tapeworm. The drug is given fasting in a dose of 1 g which is repeated in two hours, and followed by a purge. It has a toxic effect on the worm, which is killed by the drug; older remedies merely aided expulsion.

nicotinamide. A compound derived from nicotinic acid, *q.v.*, and possessing similar properties, but differs in that it has little vasodilator action. It is useful in deficiency states when the vasodilator action of nicotinic acid limits the dose.

nicotinic acid (niacin). An essential food factor, occurring in yeast, liver, etc., but now prepared synthetically. It is a specific in the treatment of pellagra. It causes vasodilation, and is used in chilblains, headache, angina pectoris. In large doses it lowers the blood cholesterol level. Daily prophylactic dose 15 to 30 mg. Daily therapeutic dose 50 to 250 mg.

nicoumalone. A synthetic anticoagulant similar to phenindione, *q.v.* Initial dose 8 to 16 mg; subsequent doses are based on the response, as shown by determination of the blood prothrombin levels.

nifuratel. An antiprotozoal agent used in the treatment of infections due to *Trichomonas vaginalis*. Dose 200 mg three times a day for seven days. Pessaries of 250 mg are also used.

nikethamide. A centrally acting respiratory stimulant with mild vasoconstrictor properties. Dose as injection of nikethamide (25%) 2 to 4 ml, by intramuscular or intravenous injection.

Nilevar. Norethandrolone, q.v.

niridazole. Valuable in the treatment of schistosomiasis, and also used in amoebiasis. Side-effects include nausea, anxiety and confusion. Dose 500 mg to 1·5 g daily.

nitrazepam. An hypnotic of low toxicity that has a more selective action than the barbiturates. May be of value in insomnia as an alternative to more toxic drugs, as even excessive overdose has few serious effects. Dose 5 to 10 mg.

nitrofurantoin. A urinary antiseptic with a wide range of activity. It is of value in renal infections that have become resistant to other forms of treatment. Average dose 100 mg four times a day. Often used in rotation with other urinary antiseptics. Peripheral neuritis has occurred after extended treatment.

nitrofurazone. A wide-range antibacterial compound used mainly for infected wounds and preparation for skin graft-ing. Sensitization may occur after continuous application. Occasionally used orally in the treatment of trypanosomiasis in doses of 1 to 2 g daily.

Nitrogen mustard. Mustine, q.v.

nitrous oxide. The oldest inhalation anaesthetic, once known as laughing gas. Supplied in blue cylinders, it is widely used for brief operative work, and for induction.

Nivaquine. Chloroquine, q.v.

Nobrium. Medazepam, q.v.

Noludar. Methyprylone, q.v.

Nolvadex. Tamoxifen, q.v.

noradrenaline. One of the hormones of the adrenal gland. It raises blood-pressure mainly by a general vasoconstriction, whereas adrenaline increases the blood pressure by constricting the peripheral vessels and increasing the cardiac output. Given by slow intravenous injection in the treatment of shock, peripheral failure, and low blood-pressure states, but the response may fluctuate with small variations in dose. Ampoules containing 4 mg are available, and the dose is based on the patient's need and response. Care must be taken to avoid extra-venous injection.

norethandrolone. A steroid compound related to testosterone, with similar tissue-building or anabolic properties, but with a markedly reduced virilizing action. It can therefore be used for its protein-building properties in both sexes in convalescence, in wasting diseases, osteoporosis and senile debility. Dose 10 to 20 mg orally; 25 mg by injection.

norethisterone. An orally active drug with a progesterone-like action in inhibiting ovulation. Used in amenorrhoea and functional uterine bleeding. Dose 5 to 20 mg daily. In lower doses in association with small doses of an oestrogen, norethisterone and related drugs are in wide use as oral contraceptives.

Norflex. Orphenadrine, *q.v.*

nortriptyline. A psychotherapeutic drug with a specific antidepressant action similar to that of imipramine, *q.v.* May be used in association with a chlorpromazine-type drug if the depression is associated with anxiety and agitation. Dose 20 to 75 mg daily.

novobiocin. An orally active antibiotic derived from *Streptomyces spheroides.* The range of activity includes both Gram-positive and Gram-negative organisms, but its value is limited by the rapid appearance of resistant bacteria. Yellow pigmentation of the skin may be observed

during treatment. Dose 250 mg six-hourly, increased in severe infections.

Noxyflex. A derivative of urea with marked antibacterial and antifungal properties. Used as a 1 to 2·5% solution for irrigation and topically as a spray. When used for bladder instillation, the addition of an anaesthetic is necessary to relieve the intense burning sensation.

Numotac. Isoetharine, *q.v.*

Nupercaine. Cinchocaine, *q.v.*

nux vomica. The seeds from which strychnine, *q.v.*, is obtained.

Nydrane. Beclamide, *q.v.*

Nystan. Nystatin, *q.v.*

nystatin. A fungicidal antibiotic, used in the prophylaxis and treatment of intestinal and vaginal moniliasis. Oral tablets contain 500,000 units, pessaries contain 100,000 units. It has no significant action against intestinal bacteria.

O

Oblivon. Methylpentynol, *q.v.*

oestradiol. The oestrogenic hormone controlling ovulation and menstruation. Given in oestrogen deficiency, such as menopause, kraurosis, amenorrhoea, etc. Also used in malignant disease of the breast and prostate. Dose 1 to

10 mg. For injections, oestradiol monobenzoate is preferred. Dose 1 to 5 mg daily, intramuscularly.

Omnopon. A preparation of opium alkaloids similar to papaveretum, q.v.

Oncovin. Vincristine, q.v.

Operidine. Phenoperidine, q.v.

Opilon. Thymoxamine, q.v.

opium. The dried juice from the capsules of the opium poppy, and occurs as a brown powder containing 10% of morphine. The action of opium is mainly that of its principal constituent, morphine, but the other alkaloids present modify the action, and opium is preferred to morphine when a constipating action is required, as in intestinal disorders. Opium preparations include tincture of opium or laudanum (dose 0·3 to 2 ml); paregoric or camphorated tincture of opium (dose 2 to 4 ml). Dose of opium 30 to 200 mg.

Opticrom. A preparation of sodium cromoglycate, q.v., used for vernal conjunctivitis.

Oradexon. Dexamethasone, q.v.

Orap, Pimozide, q.v.

Orbenin. Cloxacillin, q.v.

orciprenaline. A bronchodilator similar to isoprenaline, q.v.

orphenadrine. A spasmolytic drug, used in the treatment of parkinsonism, and for the relief of voluntary muscle

spasm. Dose 200 to 400 mg daily in divided doses.

Orudis. Ketoprofen, q.v.

Ospolot. Sulthiame, q.v.

ouabain (strophanthin-G). A cardiac drug similar to strophanthin-K, but twice as active. Dose 0·12 to 0·25 mg as a single intravenous injection. See also strophanthus.

oxazepam. An anxiolytic agent useful in agitation, tension and anxiety. Dose 15 mg daily, doubled if required.

oxolinic acid. Has bactericidal properties chiefly against Gram-negative organisms. Of value in acute and recurrent infections of the urinary tract. Dose 750 mg twice daily. May cause gastric disturbance and C.N.S. stimulation. Not for use in pregnancy.

oxprenolol. An adrenergic blocking agent similar in action and use to propranolol, q.v. Oral dose 40 mg initially, rising to 200 mg or more daily; 1 to 2 mg by intravenous injection.

Oxycel. Oxidized cellulose in the form of woven gauze strips. Has haemostatic properties, and if left in a closed wound it is eventually absorbed.

oxymetholone. A steroid compound related to testosterone, and with similar anabolic or protein-building properties. In oxymetholone, and in related steroids, the anabolic effects have been largely separated from the androgen or virilizing effects, thus permitting their use in female patients and children. These drugs are therefore useful in metabolic disturbance after operation, in convalescence, osteoporosis and anorexia. Dose 5 to 30 mg daily.

oxypertine. A tranquillizer used in anxiety neuroses, psychoses and withdrawn schizophrenic states. Dose 10 to 40 mg in mild conditions, up to 300 mg daily in schizophrenia.

oxyphenbutazone. A derivative of phenylbutazone, with similar analgesic and anti-inflammatory properties. Also used locally as eye ointment. Dose 300 to 600 mg daily initially, maintenance doses not more than 400 mg daily. The drug should be discontinued if a favourable response does not occur in four to five days.

oxytetracycline. An antibiotic derived from cultures of *Streptomyces rimosus*. Has a very wide range of activity against many organisms, including some viruses, and is useful in penicillin-resistant conditions. Usually given orally, but intramuscular and intravenous preparations are available. Intravenous injections must be given slowly in dilute solution to avoid thrombosis. Average adult dose 250 mg six-hourly. Side-effects, including gastro-intestinal disturbances and rectal irritation, may occur if treatment is prolonged.

oxytocin. The oxytocic fraction of pituitary extract, *q.v.* Used mainly in post-partum haemorrhage, as when used for induction of labour the response may lead to severe uterine contractions. Dose 2 to 5 units by subcutaneous or intramuscular injection.

P

P.A.S. Para-aminosalicylic acid, *q.v.*

P.I.D. Phenindione, *q.v.*

Pacitron. Tryptophan, *q.v.*

Palfium. Dextromoramide, *q.v.*

Paludrine. Proguanil, *q.v.*

Panadol. Paracetamol, *q.v.*

pancreatin. A preparation containing the pancreatic enzymes, trypsin, lipase and amylase. Used to aid digestion in pancreatic disease. Dose 0·5 to 1 g.

pancuronium. A muscle-relaxant similar to tubocurarine, *q.v.*, but with the advantage that it has no histamine-releasing or cardiovascular action. Dose: 2 to 4 mg intravenously initially, with 2 mg supplements as required.

pantothenic acid. A constituent

of the vitamin B complex. Its significance in human nutrition is still unknown. Dose 100 mg or more daily.

papaveretum. A preparation of the alkaloids of opium, containing approximately 50% of morphine. Used mainly by injection, often in association with hyoscine (scopolamine). Dose 10 to 15 mg.

papaverine. One of the alkaloids of opium. It has little analgesic action, and is used mainly as a smooth muscle relaxant in peripheral vascular diseases, spasm and asthma. Dose 60 to 300 mg orally, 30 to 100 mg by intramuscular or intravenous injection.

para-aminosalicylic acid. This compound has a bacteriostatic action on the tubercle bacillus, and is widely used in tuberculous disease. As the drug is rapidly absorbed and eliminated, frequent doses are necessary to maintain adequate blood-levels. It should be prescribed in association with at least one other antitubercular drug to inhibit the emergence of drug-resistant strains of bacteria. Dose 10 to 15 g daily in divided doses.

paracetamol. A mild analgesic derived from phenacetin, *q.v.* It has the general properties of the parent drug, but fewer side-effects. Dose 0·5 to 1 g.

Paradione. Paramethadione, *q.v.*

paraffin. A generic name for hydrocarbon mixtures. Soft paraffin is the common ointment base; liquid paraffin is a lubricant laxative. Hard paraffin is used in the wax bath treatment of rheumatic conditions.

paraformaldehyde. A solid form of formaldehyde; used for sterilizing catheters, disinfecting rooms, etc., by vaporization.

paraldehyde. A colourless liquid with strong characteristic odour. It is a rapid-acting sedative similar in effect to chloral, but less depressant. Given orally, or intramuscularly, and may be given rectally after dilution with arachis oil. Dose 5 to 10 ml orally, or by intramuscular injection; 15 to 30 ml rectally.

paramethadione. An anticonvulsant similar to troxidone, *q.v.*, and useful in petit mal that does not respond to that drug. Dose 900 to 1,800 mg daily.

Parathormone. A solution of the hormones of the parathyroid gland controlling the calcium level of the blood. Given in early treatment of tetany due to parathyroid deficiency. Dose 20 to 30 units by intramuscular injection.

parathyroid. The small glands associated with the thyroid, controlling calcium metabolism. Their removal causes tetany which may be treated immediately with Parathormone, followed by calcium gluconate and A.T. 10.

Pardolel. Bromocriptine, *q.v.*

paregoric. Camphorated tincture of opium. A constituent of Gee's Linctus and many other cough preparations. Dose 2 to 4 ml.

pargyline. A monoamine oxidase inhibitor used in the treatment of benign hypertension. It also has mild, central stimulant properties, and may influence mood. Dose 10 to 50 mg or more daily, according to response.

Parnate. Tranylcypromine, *q.v.*

Pavulon. Pancuronium, *q.v.*

Peganone. An anticonvulsant sometimes used with phenytoin in epilepsy not responding to other drugs. Dose up to 2 g daily.

pempidine. A ganglion-blocking agent used like mecamylamine, *q.v.*, in the treatment of hypertension. Dose 2·5 to 7·5 mg initially, subsequently increased according to response.

Penbritin. Ampicillin, *q.v.*

penicillamine. A breakdown product of penicillin, which has the power of combining with certain metals to form a water-soluble, non-toxic complex that is excreted in the urine. It is used in Wilson's disease, which is due to the retention of copper in the body, and in poisoning by lead and mercury. Also used in rheumatoid arthritis no longer responding to other treatment. Dose 0·25 to 1·5 g daily.

penicillin, benzyl penicillin, penicillin G. The first of the antibiotics, *q.v.* It is well tolerated and is widely used in the treatment of infections due to Gram-positive organisms and the spirochaetes of syphilis and yaws, but the efficacy varies widely according to the sensitivity of the organisms to the drug. Penicillin is usually given by intramuscular injection, and as it is rapidly excreted the action is relatively brief, but derivatives are available, such as procaine-penicillin, which have a longer action. Penicillin V is an orally active derivative. The dose of penicillin varies considerably according to need and response, but an average dose of soluble penicillin is 500,000 units; of procaine-penicillin 300,000 units; of penicillin V, 125 to 250 mg. Methicillin, *q.v.*, cloxacillin, *q.v.*, and flucloxacillin, *q.v.* are derivatives of penicillin active against resistant *staphylococci*; ampicillin is a derivative with a wide range of activity against Gram-positive and Gram-negative organisms; carbenicillin, *q.v.*, is active against *Pseudomonas pyocyanea*.

pentamidine isethionate. A synthetic drug used in trypanosomiasis and other tropical diseases. Dose 150 to 300 mg by intramuscular or intravenous injection.

pentazocine. A powerful analgesic of the morphine type, but free from addictive properties, although dependence may occur with long treatment. Dose 25 to 100 mg orally, every three to four hours, 20 to 60 mg by intramuscular injection.

pentobarbitone sodium. A short-acting barbiturate, given orally in doses of 100 to 200 mg for insomnia. Doses of 250 to 500 mg intravenously as an anticonvulsant.

pentolinium. A ganglionic blocking agent once used in the treatment of hypertension. Still used occasionally in diagnosis and to assess response.

Pentothal. Thiopentone sodium, *q.v.*

peppermint oil. Aromatic carminative. Widely used as peppermint water as a flavouring agent in mixtures.

Peptavlon. A synthetic compound which resembles natural gastrin in its ability to

stimulate gastric secretion. It is given in doses of 6 mg per kg body-weight by subcutaneous injection to test gastric secretory ability. It is less likely to cause the side-effects of histamine gastric tests.

Percorten. Deoxycortone, *q.v.*

Periactin. Cyproheptadine, *q.v.*

pericyazine. A tranquillizer of the chlorpromazine type, used mainly in schizophrenia and severe anxiety states. dose 10 to 25 mg or more, according to need.

Peroidin. Tablets of potassium perchlorate (50 mg and 200 mg). Used in hyperthyroidism and thyrotoxicosis as an alternative to carbimazole, *q.v.* Dose 200 mg, four times a day for one month, subsequently reduced by half or less according to need.

perphenazine. A derivative of chlorpromazine, used for similar purposes, but effective in lower doses. Tablets of 2, 4 and 8 mg, ampoules of 5 mg.

Pertofran. Desipramine, *q.v.*

pethidine. A synthetic analgesic with spasmolytic properties. Widely employed as an alternative to morphine for pre- and post-operative use. Of value in obstetrics as it has a less depressant action than morphine on the respiration. Dose 25 to 100 mg orally, or by intramuscular injection; 25 to 50 mg intravenously.

Pethilorfan. A mixture of pethidine and levallorphan. The latter is a narcotic antagonist, and in suitable doses it is said to reduce the respiratory depression caused by pethidine without reducing the analgesic effect.

Perolysen. Pempidine, *q.v.*

Phanodorm. Cyclobarbitone, *q.v.*

phemitone. Sedative with anticonvulsant properties. Given in epilepsy as a less toxic alternative to phenobarbitone. Dose 60 to 200 mg.

phenacetin. A mild analgesic and antipyretic. It has been widely used, as toxic effects after standard doses are uncommon. Prolonged treatment in full doses may cause kidney damage and it has now been largely replaced by paracetamol, *q.v.* Dose 300 to 600 mg.

phenazocine. A synthetic morphine-like drug, with similar analgesic properties, but with a more rapid and longer action, and effective in smaller doses. Dose 5 mg orally; 2 to 4 mg by intramuscular injection, 1 to 2 mg intravenously.

phenazone. A synthetic analgesic similar to phenacetin. Present in combination with chloral in Welldorm, *q.v.*

phenazopyridine. A urinary analgesic, useful in relieving the pain of cystitis and related conditions. Dose 200 mg.

Phenergan. Promethazine, *q.v.*

phenethicillin. A penicillin derivative that is effective orally, giving blood-levels comparable with those following injections of penicillin. Indicated in infections due to penicillin-sensitive organisms, and in some resistant staphylococcal infections. Dose: 125 to 500 mg.

phenformin. An oral hypoglycaemic drug, unrelated to tolbutamide, and may be effective when tolbutamide has failed to lower the blood-sugar level. May also be given in association with other drugs. Dose 25 to 150 mg daily.

phenindamine. An antihistamine of medium potency. It differs from most antihistamines in having a mild central stimulant action, and so rarely causes drowsiness. Dose 25 to 50 mg.

phenindione. A widely employed oral anticoagulant, with a consistent and reliable action. The onset of effect is slow, and initial doses are often given in association with heparin, *q.v.*, which gives immediate anticoagulant cover before the effects of phenindione can be anticipated.

Initial dose 200 to 300 mg, maintenance doses 25 to 100 mg daily.

phenobarbitone. A powerful sedative, hypnotic and anticonvulsant drug. It has the general properties of the long-acting barbiturates, and is widely used in epilepsy, often with phenytoin, *q.v.* Dose 30 to 125 mg.

phenobarbitone sodium. The soluble form of phenobarbitone, *q.v.*, having a more rapid action. Used mainly by intramuscular injection. Dose 30 to 125 mg; up to 200 mg as a single dose by intramuscular injection.

phenol (carbolic acid). One of the early antiseptics, but now little used. Present in Calamine Lotion, as weak solutions have an antipruritic action.

phenolphthalein. A white insoluble tasteless powder, used as a purgative. It is often given with emulsion of liquid paraffin. Dose 50 to 300 mg.

phenolsulphonphthalein. A red compound used by intravenous injection as a test of renal function. In health, at least 50% of the test dose will be excreted in the urine one hour after the injection. Dose 6 mg by intravenous injection.

phenoperidine. A morphine-like analgesic, often used in association with droperidol, *q.v.* Dose 0·5 to 5 mg by intravenous injection.

phenoxybenzamine. A peripheral vasodilator, used in Raynaud's disease, vasospasm, and to control the hypertension caused by phaeochromocytoma. Dose 10 to 20 mg by intravenous injection, increasing according to need and response.

phensuximide. An anticonvulsant used in petit mal epilepsy. Of value in patients not responding to other drugs. Dose 1 g daily, increasing to 3 g daily in divided doses if necessary.

phentolamine. An adrenolytic drug which can temporarily reverse the action of adrenaline and noradrenaline on the blood-vessels. Used mainly in the diagnosis of phaeochromocytoma, and also to control the blood-pressure during surgical removal of the tumour. Dose 5 to 10 mg, by intravenous or intramuscular injection.

phenylbutazone. An analgesic used mainly in treatment of rheumatic and arthritic conditions. Relief of pain is usually rapid, although inflammatory swelling is reduced less quickly. Also useful in the treatment of gout. Gastric disturbance is not uncommon and mucosal ulceration, rash and blood disorders may occur. Blood counts during treatment are necessary. The dose should be reduced to a low maintenance level as soon as relief is obtained. Dose 200 to 400 mg daily in divided doses.

phenylephrine. A powerful vasoconstrictor similar to adrenaline, but less toxic and suitable for use during anaesthesia. Given for its pressor effect in doses of 1 to 5 mg by intramuscular injection. It is also used locally as 1:400 solution as nasal decongestive, and as eye-drops, 0·1 to 10%.

phenylmercuric nitrate. A mercurial antibacterial and antifungal agent. Used in antifungal creams; occasionally as a lotion or for irrigation in strengths of 1 in 10,000 or less.

phenytoin sodium. An anticonvulsant used in epilepsy of the grand mal type. It has little hypnotic effect and combined treatment with phenobarbitone may evoke the best response. May cause skin rashes, dizziness, gastric disturbances, etc., and in a few cases marked overgrowth of gums. Dose 50 to 100 mg thrice daily.

pholcodine. Closely resembles codeine in its selective depressant action on the cough centre, but it has no analgesic action. It is present in a range of products used for the relief of useless cough, and has the advantage over codeine of not causing constipation. Dose 5 to 15 mg.

Phospholine Iodide. A powerful and long-acting miotic drug, used in the treatment of glaucoma. The strength (0·06 to 0·25%) and frequency of use depend on the individual response.

phthalylsulphathiazole. A poorly absorbed sulphonamide used in gastro-intestinal infections, and for pre- and post-operative use in abdominal surgery. Dose 5 to 10 g daily in divided doses.

Physeptone. Methadone, *q.v.*

physostigmine. The alkaloid of calabar beans, used as miotic (0·25 to 1%) to counteract effects of atropine, and in the treatment of glaucoma. Solutions may turn pink on storage.

picrotoxin. A powerful central nervous system stimulant, which has been used in the treatment of barbiturate poisoning. Given by intravenous injection in doses of 3 to 6 mg.

pilocarpine. Resembles physostigmine, and is used as a miotic in glaucoma as 0·5 to 2% solution.

pimozide. A tranquillizer of value in schizophrenia, as it controls the delusions without causing drowsiness. Not effective in mania or hyperactivity. Dose 2 to 4 mg initially as a single dose, increasing to 10 mg daily.

Pipanol. Benzhexol, *q.v.*

piperazine. An effective anthelmintic against threadworms and roundworms. Available as elixir and tablets. Dose 500 mg twice a day (4 to 6 years), up to 1 g twice a day (14 years and over). Seven days' treatment is usually sufficient. For roundworms a single dose of up to 4 g is given, according to age. The worms are narcotized, and eliminated in the faeces, so a purge may be necessary to ensure expulsion of the worms before the effects of the drug disappear.

piritamide. A powerful analgesic used in the relief of post-operative pain. Not suitable for prolonged use as it may cause dependence. Dose 20 mg by intramuscular injection.

Piriton. Chlorpheniramine, *q.v.*

Pitocin. Oxytocin, *q.v.*

Pitressin. Vasopressin, *q.v.*

pituitary extract. An aqueous extract of the posterior lobe of the pituitary gland. It has been used to check postpartum haemorrhage by inducing adequate contraction of the uterus, but oxytocin, *q.v.*, is now preferred. Also used by injection, or as a snuff, for its anti-diuretic effects in the treatment of diabetes insipidus. Dose 0·2 to 1 ml (2 to 10 units) by subcutaneous or intramuscular injection.

podophyllum resin. A powerful purgative, usually given with carminatives to prevent griping, also used as paint (25% in liquid paraffin) to remove condylomata.

poldine. A synthetic atropine-like substance with a marked inhibitory action on gastric secretion. Used in hyperacidity and gastric ulcer. Dose 2 to 4 mg.

polidexide. A compound that indirectly lowers the blood level of cholesterol by inhibiting the absorption of bile acids from the intestines. Used in the treatment of hypercholesterolaemia. Dose 3 g. May also decrease the absorption of certain drugs, such as anticoagulants and some antibiotics.

polymyxin B. An antibiotic obtained from *Bacillus polymyxa*, and of value in infections due to *Ps. pyocyanea* and other Gram-negative bacteria. Kidney damage and other toxic effects may limit its systemic use and value. Dose 250,000 units four-hourly by intramuscular injection. Also used for topical application, often in association with hydrocortisone.

Polymyxin E. Colistin, *q.v.*

Ponderax. Fenfluramine, *q.v.*

Ponstan. Mefenamic acid, *q.v.*

potassium bromide. Once used as a sedative, but now virtually obsolete. Overdosage, usually due to self-medication, is still occasionally seen, manifested by mental dullness, drowsiness and rash.

potassium chloride. A constituent of Darrow's and other electrolyte replacement injection solutions. Is often given orally to replace the potassium loss that may occur during treatment with chlorothiazide or related diuretics. Such potassium loss may cause muscle weakness and cardiac arrhythmias. In severe deficiency, potassium chloride can be given intravenously, but dose and rate of administration require care, as in excess, potassium can cause cardiac arrest.

potassium citrate. An alkaline diuretic excreted in the urine as bicarbonate. It is useful in cystitis and other inflammatory conditions of the urinary tract where the urine is acid; in gout, to increase the excretion of uric acid, and during sulphonamide therapy to prevent crystalluria. Dose 1 to 2 g.

potassium iodide. It reduces the viscosity of bronchial mucus, and is used as an expectorant; it is of value in the prophylaxis and treatment of simple goitre which is due to a deficiency of iodide. Also given pre-operatively in thyrotoxicosis, as it alters the texture of the gland, and facilitates surgery. Dose as an expectorant 250 to 500 mg, in thyrotoxicosis 30 to 60 mg.

potassium permanganate. Purple crystals, soluble in water. A powerful oxidizing and deodorizing agent, used 1:1,000 as lotion, 1:10,000 to 1:5,000 as mouthwash, douche, bladder washout and bath.

practolol. A drug similar in action to propranolol, *q.v.* Ocular and other side-effects have been observed after long use, and the drug is now available only in hospitals.

prazosin. A drug with a specific relaxant action on arteriolar smooth muscle. It produces a slow and sustained fall in blood-pressure with few haemodynamic side-effects. Claimed to be of value in all grades of benign hypertension. Dose 2 mg three times a day initially, adjusted after 4 to 6 weeks.

prednisolone. A derivative of hydrocortisone, with actions, uses and doses comparable with those of prednisone, *q.v.*

prednisone. A derivative of cortisone, *q.v.*, with similar properties, but effective in lower dose, and causing less sodium retention and electrolyte disturbance. Prednisone and prednisolone are widely used in a variety of unrelated conditions, including arthritis, rheumatoid conditions, inflammatory skin conditions, in allergic states, and in status asthmaticus. Large doses are sometimes given in leukaemia and other blood disorders. Prednisone is also useful in nephrotic oedema. It is also used with other drugs as an immunosuppressive agent in transplant surgery. Both prednisone and prednisolone may cause dyspepsia and peptic ulcer in susceptible patients, and for long-term suppressive treatment the dose should not exceed 8 mg daily. For initial therapy and in crisis, the dose may vary from 20 to 100 mg daily, adjusted to response as soon as the condition permits. Special products are available for intramuscular and intravenous injection; for intra-articular injection, and for local use as eye-drops. Cortisone is preferred in adrenal deficiency states where a salt-retaining effect is essential.

Predsol, Prednesol. Brand names of some prednisolone products.

Pregnyl. Chorionic gonadotrophin, *q.v.*

Pressimmune. An equine immunoglobulin preparation obtained from horses by immunization with human lymphocytes. It suppresses cell-mediated immunity, but has less influence on antibody production and resistance to bacterial infection. Used as an immunosuppressive agent in transplant surgery, after sensitivity tests.

Priadel. Lithium carbonate, *q.v.*

primidone. An anticonvulsant drug of value in the treatment of grand mal and psychomotor epilepsy, but some cases of petit mal also respond. The changeover from other forms of therapy should be gradual. Drowsiness is a not uncommon side-effect. Dose 250 mg to 2 g daily.

Primolut N. Norethisterone, *q.v.*

Primperan. Metoclopramide. *q.v.*

Pripsen. Granules containing piperazine, *q.v.*, and a senna extract, this providing an anthelmintic and a purge in a single dose of 10 g.

Priscol. Tolazoline, *q.v.*

Privine. Naphazoline, *q.v.*

Pro-banthine. Propantheline, *q.v.*

probenecid. An orally active compound that increases the excretion of uric acid, and so is useful in the treatment of gout. It is given in doses of 0·5 to 1 g daily, together with alkalis. The drug also has the reverse property of delaying the excretion of penicillin and para-amino-salicylic acid, and is given in doses of 0·5 g six-hourly to raise the blood-levels of those drugs.

procainamide. A procaine derivative occasionally of value in the treatment of cardiac arrhythmias. Dose 500 mg orally or intramuscularly, increased later to 1 g. Intravenous use in emergencies when a rapid response is essential requires care, as a marked fall in blood-pressure may occur.

procaine hydrochloride. A local anaesthetic of the cocaine type, now largely replaced by lignocaine, q.v. Solutions used vary in strength from 0·5 to 2% often with the addition of adrenaline or noradrenaline to prolong the action.

procarbazine. A cytostatic agent that inhibits cell division. Useful in Hodgkin's disease and lymphomas that no longer respond to other drugs. Dose 50 to 300 mg. Initial doses should be low to reduce nausea.

prochlorperazine. A tranquilliser and anti-emetic of the chlorpromazine type, but more powerful, and effective in lower doses. Anti-emetic dose 10 to 25 mg. Psychiatric dose 15 to 100 mg daily.

procyclidine. A spasmolytic drug similar to benzhexol, q.v., used mainly in the treatment of parkinsonism. Reduces rigidity more than tremor. Dose 7·5 to 30 mg daily in divided doses.

Prodoxol. Oxolinic acid, q.v.

progesterone. The hormone of the corpus luteum, responsible for the preparation of the uterus to receive a fertilized ovum. Used occasionally in treatment of functional uterine haemorrhage. Dose 2 to 60 mg by intramuscular injection. Orally effective drugs are now preferred.

proguanil hydrochloride. A synthetic antimalarial of high potency and low toxicity, widely used in suppressive and therapeutic treatment. Dose 100 to 300 mg daily.

promazine. Has the actions and uses of chlorpromazine, q.v. Useful in the treatment of restlessness in the aged. Dose ranges from 50 to 800 mg daily, orally, intravenously or intramuscularly.

promethazine. A long-acting antihistamine with sedative properties. Of value in urticaria, parkinsonism, and in premedication. Dose 20 to 50 mg daily, orally or by intra-muscular injection.

Prominal. Phemitone, *q.v.*

Pronestyl. Procainamide, *q.v.*

Propaderm. Beclomethasone, *q.v.*

propanidid. A short-acting intra-venous anaesthetic, unrelated to the barbiturates. Recovery is rapid and complete, with few side-effects. Dose 5 to 10 mg per kg body-weight as 5% solution.

propantheline. An atropine-like compound used as a spasmo-lytic in peptic ulcer, pyloro-spasm, ureteral spasms, etc. Side-effects include dryness of mouth and blurring of vision. Dose 15 mg.

propionic acid. Has fungicidal properties and is used in local fungus infections as oint-ment or dusting powder.

propranolol. A beta-adrenergic blocking agent that reduces the cardiac response to circu-lating adrenaline. It is of value in reducing the work load on the heart during exercise, and stress, and is used in the treat-ment of angina, coronary in-sufficiency, cardiac arrhyth-mias and hypertension. May cause bronchospasm in asth-matic patients. More cardio-selective drugs, such as ace-butolol, *q.v.*, are now avail-able. Dose 20 to 120 mg or more daily, 3 to 10 mg intra-venously.

propylthiouracil. A thyroid in-hibitor occasionally used in thyrotoxicosis. Dose 50 to 200 mg.

prostaglandin. A generic term applied to a series of closely related fatty acid derivatives, originally extracted from prostate gland, but now pre-pared synthetically. They are widely distributed in animal tissues, and have a complex and varying range of biologi-cal activity. Thus they may have a smooth-muscle stimu-lating or relaxant action, pressor, vasodilator, inflam-matory or other properties. There is evidence that the anti-inflammatory action of aspirin and related drugs may be due to an inhibition of prostaglandin synthesis. There are four main groups of prostaglandins (PGA, PGB, PGE and PGF) which can be further subdivided. PGE_2 and PGF_2 have been given by intravenous infusion in the induction of labour and in the termination of pregnancy, and an oral form is available as dinoprostone, *q.v.*

Prostigmin. Neostigmine, *q.v.*

Prostin E$_2$. Dinoprostone, *q.v.*

protamine sulphate. A simple protein obtained from fish sperm. It neutralizes the anti-coagulant effect of heparin, and it is used in controlling the haemorrhage that may occur during heparin therapy. It is given intravenously in doses of 5 ml as a 1% solution; 1 ml will neutralize about 1,000 units of heparin.

protein hydrolysate. The soluble product of the enzymatic hydrolysis of a protein such as casein. It contains essential amino-acids and purified forms are available for intravenous use. Solutions containing dextrose and alcohol are also available. Used in severe protein deficiency, and after gastric surgery.

prothionamide. A tuberculostatic drug similar to ethionamide, *q.v.* Dose: 0·75 to 1 g daily. Useful when ethionamide is not tolerated.

prothipendyl. A tranquillizing drug with actions and uses similar to those of chlorpromazine. Dose 40 to 120 mg daily.

protriptyline. An antidepressant with a rapid action, and is largely free from any sedative properties. Similar to imipramine, *q.v.*, in action, but if anxiety or tension is also present, it may be given with tranquillizers. Dose 15 to 60 mg daily.

Pularin. Heparin, *q.v.*

Puri-Nethol. Mercaptopurine, *q.v.*

Pyopen. Carbenicillin, *q.v.*

pyrazinamide. A tuberculostatic drug used in infections resistant to standard treatment. Can be given alone for short periods, but for long treatment combined therapy is essential. May cause liver damage and hyperuricaemia. Dose 20 to 35 mg per kg body-weight daily in divided doses.

Pyridium. Phenazopyridine, *q.v.*

pyridostigmine. An anticholinesterase similar to neostigmine, but with a slower and more prolonged action. Useful in myasthenia gravis and paralytic ileus. Dose 60 to 240 mg orally, 1 to 5 mg by intramuscular injection.

pyridoxine (vitamin B_6). This vitamin plays an essential part in protein metabolism. Apart from deficiency states, it has been used in alcoholism, muscular dystrophy, agranulocytosis, nausea and vomiting of pregnancy. Dose 20 to 100 mg.

pyrimethamine. An anti-malarial drug similar to proguanil, but its chief value is in prophylaxis. Regular use will inhibit most relapses of benign tertian malaria. Dose 25 to 50 mg weekly.

pyroxylin. Nitrated cellulose. When dissolved in alcohol and ether, it is the basis of collodion, *q.v.*

Q

Quinacrine. Mepacrine, *q.v.*

quinalbarbitone sodium. A short-acting barbiturate with an effect that persists from two to four hours. Used in mild insomnia and anxiety states. Dose 50 to 200 mg.

quinidine. An alkaloid of cinchona, similar to quinine, but it has a valuable, specific depressant effect on the auricle muscle. It has been used in the treatment of early atrial fibrillation and in paroxysmal tachycardia, but beta-adrenergic blocking agents, *q.v.*, are often preferred. Quinidine may cause tinnitus and other side-effects in sensitive patients, and a test dose of 200 mg is often given. If tolerated, a dose of 300 mg may be given three to five times a day, reduced later if normal rhythm is resumed. Treatment should be stopped if response does not occur within 10 days.

quinine. The principal alkaloid of cinchona bark. It is still used in some areas for the treatment of malaria, but synthetic antimalarials such as chloroquine and proguanil are now preferred. Dose 60 to 600 mg. Prolonged use or overdose causes cinchonism, a syndrome of nausea, tinnitus, headache and rash.

R

Rastinon. Tolbutamide, *q.v.*

Rauwiloid. A mixture of alkaloids of rauwolfia. The action is basically that of the main constituent, reserpine, *q.v.*

rauwolfia. The dried roots of *Rauwolfia serpentina*. Used in the treatment of hypertension because of its depressant action on the central nervous system. The action is mainly that of its chief alkaloid, reserpine, *q.v.* Dose 200 mg daily initially, maintenance dose 50 to 300 mg daily.

Redeptin. Fluspirilene, *q.v.*

Redoxon. Ascorbic acid, *q.v.*

reserpine. The principal alkaloid of rauwolfia, *q.v.* It is used in mild hypertension, but a fall in blood-pressure occurs only after continued treatment, although subjective improvement may occur earlier. Also used for its sedative action in mild anxiety states and chronic psychoses. Dose in hypertension 0·1 to 0·5 mg daily; in psychiatric conditions doses up to 5 mg daily have been given. These higher doses may cause severe depression, nasal congestion and gastric disturbances, and more controllable drugs are often preferred.

Resonium A. A synthetic exchange resin that can take up potassium, and is sometimes of value in the treatment of hyperkalaemia associated with surgical shock anuria and similar states. Dose 15 g orally up to four times a day.

resorcin. An antipruritic and keratolytic agent used mainly as ointment in acne, and as hair lotions for removing dandruff. Myxoedema has been reported following the prolonged use of resorcin prepartions on open areas.

Rheomacrodex. A dextran, *q.v.*, preparation used mainly to improve blood-flow and prevent 'sludging' of red cells after injury. Useful in various types of peripheral ischaemia.

rhubarb. The dried rhizome of various species of Rheum, from China and Tibet. Dose 0·2 to 1 g. Used occasionally in full doses as a mild purgative and in small doses as an astringent bitter.

riboflavine (vitamin B_2). An orange-yellow powder. It is part of the vitamin B complex, and is concerned with the oxidation of carbohydrates and amino-acids. A deficiency causes several characteristic effects, including angular stomatitis and 'burning feet'. It is given in doses of 1 to 10 mg in deficiency states associated with restricted diets or poor absorption.

Rifadin. Rifampicin, *q.v.*

rifampicin. An antibiotic used mainly with isoniazid in the treatment of tubercular infections resistant to other drugs. Dose: 450 to 600 mg as a single daily dose before breakfast.

Rimactane. Rifampicin, *q.v.*

Ringer's solution. An electrolyte replacement solution containing sodium chloride, potassium chloride and calcium chloride.

Ritalin. Methyl phenidate, *q.v.*

Roccal. Benzalkonium, *q.v.*

Rogitine. Phentolamine, *q.v.*

Rondomycin. Methacycline, *q.v.*

Ronicol. A peripheral vasodilator similar to nicotinic acid, *q.v.*, given orally or by injection in doses of 50 to 100 mg.

Rovamycin. Spiramycin, *q.v.*

rutin. A glycoside obtained from buckwheat. It has been used in the treatment of capillary fragility. Dose 20 mg. A related compound (Paroven) is used in vascular disorders of the legs in doses of 250 mg three or four times a day.

Rynacrom. Sodium cromoglycate, *q.v.*

Rythmodan. Disopyramide, *q.v.*

S

saccharin. An organic chemical with a very sweet taste, widely used as a non-calorific substitute for sugar. Has been used by rapid intravenous injection (2·5 g in 4 ml) for arm-tongue circulation time.

Salazopyrin. Sulphasalazine, *q.v.*

salbutamol. A bronchodilator similar in action to isoprenaline, *q.v.*, but with fewer side-effects. Dose 2 to 4 mg.

salicylic acid. White insoluble powder with keratolytic and fungicidal properties. Used as ointment (2·5%) for parasitic skin conditions, and as ointments and plasters (up to 40%) for corns and warts.

Saluric. Chlorothiazide, *q.v.*

santonin. An anthelmintic from flower-heads of artemisia. Once widely used against roundworms, but less toxic drugs such as piperazine, *q.v.*, are now preferred. Dose 60 to 200 mg.

Saroten. Amitriptyline, *q.v.*

Saventrine. A long-acting form of isoprenaline, *q.v.*, used mainly in heart block. Dose 30 mg.

Savlon. A mixture of cetrimide and chlorhexidine, *q.v.*, widely used as an effective and non-irritant antiseptic.

scopolamine. Hyoscine, *q.v.*

Secholex. Polidexide, *q.v.*

Seconal sodium. Quinalbarbitone sodium, *q.v.*

Sectral. Acebutolol, *q.v.*

Selora. Sodium-free salt substitute useful in salt-restricted diets.

senna. The leaves and pods of *Cassia* sp., used as a purgative. Standardized preparations of senna such as Senokot are now preferred.

Senokot. A proprietary preparation of senna from which the undesirable constituents have been largely removed. The product is standardized, and is reliable and effective. Available as granules or tablets.

Septrin. Referred to under trimethoprim, *q.v.*

Serc. Betahistine, *q.v.*

Serenace. Haloperidol, *q.v.*

Serenid-D. Oxazepam, *q.v.*

Serogan. Serum gonadotrophin, *q.v.*

serotonin. A natural substance in many body cells, which may act as a neurotransmitter in the central nervous system. A reduction in brain serotonin may be associated with depression (see tryptophan). Some allergic reactions may also be linked with the release of serotonin in sensitized cells (see cyproheptadine).

Serpasil. Reserpine, *q.v.*

serum gonadotrophin. The follicle-stimulating hormone obtained from pregnant mares' serum. Used with oestrogens in amenorrhoea and functional uterine bleeding. Dose 200 to 1,000 units by intramuscular injection.

silver nitrate. Used mainly as silver nitrate sticks (caustic points) for cauterizing warts.

Sinequan. Doxepin, *q.v.*

Sinthrome. Nicoumalone, *q.v.*

Sintisone. Prednisolone, *q.v.*

Slow-K. Tablets containing potassium chloride 600 mg in a wax base from which the drug is slowly released in the gastro-intestinal tract. Used to offset the potassium loss that may occur during diuretic treatment.

soda-lime. A mixture of calcium and sodium hydroxides, used in closed-circuit anaesthetic apparatus to remove carbon dioxide.

sodium acetrizoate. An organic iodine compound used as a contrast agent in intravenous pyelography, etc. Available in strengths of 30%, 50% and 70%.

sodium acid phosphate. An acid diuretic, often given with hexamine, *q.v.* In full doses it acts as a saline purgative. Dose 2 to 4 g.

sodium aminosalicylate. Sodium salt of para-amino-salicylic acid, *q.v.*

sodium aurothiomalate. A gold compound used in the treatment of active rheumatoid arthritis. It is of no value in other forms of the disease, or where deformity has already occurred. Given by intramuscular injection in doses of 10 mg weekly initially, slowly increasing to 50 mg weekly. The total dose during a course should not exceed 500 mg. Side-effects are common, and may be severe. Contraindicated in renal and hepatic disease, blood dyscrasia and hypertension.

sodium benzoate. When given by injection, it is excreted as hippuric acid, and the rate of excretion is sometimes used as an indication of liver function.

sodium bicarbonate. A widely used soluble antacid, often used in association with less soluble antacids such as magnesium carbonate or trisilicate. Dose 1 to 4 g. Also given intravenously in acidosis as 5 to 8·4% solution.

sodium chloride. An important constituent of blood and tissues. Widely used by intravenous injection as normal saline (0·9%) or as dextrose saline in treatment of dehydration and shock. Has been given orally as replacement therapy in Addison's disease; occasionally useful as an emetic in the treatment of poisoning. Used externally as saline solution as a simple cleansing lotion.

sodium citrate. An alkaline diuretic similar to potassium citrate, *q.v.*, and given for similar purposes. Dose 1 to 4 g. For citrating milk to prevent large curds, 100 mg to each feed may be used.

sodium cromoglycate. A compound with a specific effect in blocking the release of histamine and other spasmogens that cause bronchospasm and asthma in sensitized patients. Used for the prophylactic treatment of allergic asthma by inhalation with a 'Spinhaler'. Dose 20 mg. Available together with isoprenaline for the patient who finds inhalation of the simple product too irritant. Special preparations are available for use in allergic rhinitis.

sodium fusidate. An antibiotic used mainly in staphylococcal infections resistant to other drugs. Sometimes given in association with penicillin. Dose 500 mg eight-hourly with food. In severe infections it may be given by intravenous drip infusion in doses of 500 mg.

sodium lactate. Used by intravenous drip infusion in the treatment of acidosis as a $\frac{1}{6}$ molar solution, or as Hartmann's solution, q.v.

sodium perborate. White powder soluble in water, with antiseptic and deodorant properties similar to hydrogen peroxide.

sodium propionate. A mild antiseptic and fungicide. Used in ocular infections as drops (10%) and ointment (5%); in superficial fungal diseases— as ointment, jelly (10%) and pessaries.

sodium salicylate. A soluble analgesic and anti-inflammatory agent similar in action to aspirin, q.v. Used mainly in acute rheumatic fever in doses of 10 g or more daily. Such doses may cause tinnitus and nausea. Other side-effects are similar to those of aspirin.

sodium valproate. An anticonvulsant, often effective in the major forms of epilepsy. Care is necessary if given with similar drugs. Adult dose 200 mg twice daily initially, increased as required to 800 to 1400 mg daily.

sodium sulphate (Glauber's salt). A popular saline purgative. Dose 2 to 15 g. Also used as a lotion (25%) to promote drainage of infected wounds. Has been given intravenously in severe hypercalcaemia.

sodium versenate. An organic compound that combines with metals to form soluble non-toxic complexes. Used as 0·4% solution, to dissolve calcium in lime burns of the eye, and reduce corneal opacity. Occasionally given by intravenous drip infusion in hypercalcaemia.

Soframycin. Framycetin, q.v.

Soneryl. Butobarbitone, q.v.

Sotacor. Sotalol, q.v.

sotalol. A beta-adrenergic blocking agent, q.v., that is of value in the treatment of hypertension. It produces a smooth reduction in blood-pressure, largely by reducing cardiac output, and the response is not markedly influenced by exercise. Dose 80 mg initially, increasing as required to 240 to 600 mg daily in divided doses. Care is necessary in heart block and bronchial disease, and in diabetes.

Sparine. Promazine, *q.v.*

spiramycin. An orally active antibiotic effective against Gram-positive organisms. The antibacterial range resembles that of erythromycin. Dose 500 mg six-hourly.

spironolactone. A diuretic that antagonizes the action of aldosterone, *q.v.*, on the distal tubule. It increases the excretion of sodium, but reduces the excretion of potassium. Of value in oedema due to excessive secretion of aldosterone by the adrenal cortex, and resistant to the thiazide diuretics. Dose 25 mg may be given in association with other diuretics.

starch. Carbohydrate granules obtained from maize, rice, wheat or potato. Widely used as absorbent dusting powder with zinc oxide and boric acid.

Steclin. Tetracycline, *q.v.*

Stelazine. Trifluoperazine, *q.v.*

Stemetil. Prochlorperazine, *q.v.*

stibophen. A complex antimony compound, less toxic than tartar emetic, *q.v.* Used for schistosomiasis as injection of stibophen (6·4%), intramuscularly or intravenously. Dose 1·5 to 5 ml.

stilboestrol. A synthetic oestrogen, active orally, and of value in menopausal conditions and for the suppression of lactation. Dose 0·1 to 5 mg. It is also useful in the treatment of prostatic carcinoma, when very large doses may be required. Fosfesterol, *q.v.*, or stilboestrol diphosphate, has a more intense and localized effect in such carcinomas. Dose 500 mg intravenously, 100 to 200 mg orally.

stramonium. Dried leaves, similar to belladonna, containing hyoscyamine and atropine. Has been used in bronchitis and parkinsonism.

streptokinase, streptodornase. Enzymes obtained from cultures of haemolytic streptococci. They have the property of liquefying purulent exudates, blood clots, etc., and are used to clean foul wounds, pressure sores, etc. Streptokinase has been given by intrathecal injection in meningitis to break down fibrin deposits.

streptomycin. An antibiotic obtained from *Streptomyces griseus*. It is active against many organisms, and although occasionally used in urinary infections, and with penicillin in mixed infections, it is used chiefly in tuberculosis. Drug resistance may develop rapidly, so combined treatment with isoniazid, *q.v.*, and other drugs is essential. Toxic effects such as vertigo and deafness may follow high doses. Cutaneous sensitization may follow contact of the drug or its solutions with the skin. The drug is not absorbed orally, and is occasionally given by mouth in intestinal infections. Dose: up to 1 g daily by intramuscular injection; up to 100 mg by intrathecal injection; up to 1 g six-hourly orally.

strophanthus. Has cardiac properties similar to digitalis. Used mainly by intravenous injection as strophanthin-K or as ouabain, *q.v.*

strychnine. The alkaloid of nux vomica, *q.v.* It has a very bitter taste, hence it is used occasionally as gastric tonic, but has no other therapeutic value. Dose as Tincture of Nux Vomica, 0·6 to 2 ml.

Stugeron. Cinnarizine, *q.v.*

Sublimaze. Fentanyl, *q.v.*

succinylsuphathiazole. A poorly-absorbed sulphonamide used in gastro-intestinal infections, and for pre- and post-operative use in abdominal surgery. Dose 10 to 20 g daily.

sulfametopyrazine. A long-acting drug with the general antibacterial properties of the sulphonamides. Dose: 2 g once a week.

Sulfasuxidine. Succinylsulphathiazole, *q.v.*

sulphacetamide. A sulphonamide occasionally used in urinary infections. Dose 0·5 to 1 g four times a day. Sulphacetamide soluble is used as eye-drops (10 to 30%) and as ointment (2·5 to 10%).

sulphadiazine. One of the more active and less toxic sulphonamides; effective against streptococci, meningococci and many other organisms. Initial dose 3 g, followed by 1 to 1·5 g four-hourly. Given intravenously as sulphadiazine sodium in severe infections such as meningococcal meningitis.

sulphadimethoxine. A long-acting sulphonamide, effective in a wide range of infections due to sulphonamide-sensitive organisms, especially staphylococci. Dose 1 to 2 g initially, followed by 0·5 g daily.

sulphadimidine. One of the most useful and least toxic of the sulphonamides. Crystalluria and renal complications are rare, and the drug is particularly suitable for children. Initial dose 3 g; followed by six-hourly maintenance doses of 1·5 g. Smaller maintenance doses of 1 g may be adequate in urinary infections. Sulphadimidine soluble is suitable for intravenous or deep intramuscular injection.

sulphafurazole. A sulphonamide compound of particular value in urinary infections, owing to its high solubility in urine. Initial dose 3 g followed by 1 to 1·5 g, four- or six-hourly.

sulphaguanidine. A sulphonamide used in gastrointestinal infections. Now largely replaced by phthalyl- and succinylsulphathiazole. Dose 6 to 20 g daily.

sulphamerazine. A sulphonamide resembling sulphadiazine in activity, but the slower excretion increases the risk of crystalluria. The drug is rarely given alone, but survives in mixed sulphonamide products such as Sulphatriad, q.v.

sulphamethizole. A sulphonamide compound used in the treatment of urinary infections. The low dose is exceptional, being 100 to 200 mg, five to seven times a day, and side-effects are uncommon.

sulphamethoxazole. A long-acting sulphonamide used mainly in urinary and respiratory infections. Dose 2 g initially, followed by 1 g twice daily. Adequate fluid intake during treatment is necessary to reduce side-effects.

sulphamethoxypyridazine. A long-acting sulphonamide, used mainly for prophylaxis or the treatment of chronic urinary or systemic infections. Dose 1 g initially, then 0·5 g daily. The slow elimination may complicate the treatment of side-effects.

Sulphamezathine. Sulphadimidine, q.v.

sulphanilamide. One of the earliest 'sulpha' drugs. Now replaced by more active compounds.

sulphapyridine. A sulphonamide occasionally used empirically in doses of 0·5 g for dermatitis herpetiformis not responding to dapsone, q.v.

sulphasalazine. A sulphonamide which is said to be taken up selectively by the connective tissue of the intestines. Useful in the treatment of chronic ulcerative colitis. Dose 1 g, four to six times a day.

sulphathiazole. One of the early sulphonamides. Occasionally used in mixed products such as Sulphatriad, q.v.

Sulphatriad. Tablets of sulphadiazine, sulphathiazole and sulphamerazine. A mixture of sulphonamides is considered to reduce the overall toxic effects. Initial dose 4 tablets, then 2 tablets four-hourly.

sulphinpyrazone. A drug related to phenylbutazone, but with the selective action of increasing the excretion of uric acid, hence used in the treatment of chronic gout. Dose: 50 mg four times a day initially, increasing to 400 mg or more daily according to need and response. It is of no value in acute gout, but colchicine may be used if such attacks occur during treatment with sulphinpyrazone.

sulphur. Greenish-yellow insoluble powder once used extensively as ointment for scabies; present in many products of alleged value in acne. Laxative if taken internally. Dose 1 to 4 g.

sulthiame. An anticonvulsant of use in most epileptic conditions except petit mal. Dose 200 mg. The change from other treatment should be slow, with overlapping doses.

suramin. A complex organic chemical used in the treatment of the early stages of trypanosomiasis; of no value in later stages as it does not enter the cerebrospinal fluid. Dose 1 to 2 g, intravenously at weekly intervals for five weeks, after an initial dose of 500 mg to test tolerance.

surgical spirit. Methylated spirit for external use; it contains castor oil, methyl salicylate and other substances approved by the Board of Customs and Excise.

Surmontil. Trimipramine, q.v.

Suscardia. Isoprenaline, q.v.

Sustac. A long-acting preparation of glyceryl trinitrate, q.v.

suxamethonium. A short-acting muscle relaxant, with an action lasting three to five minutes. A preliminary injection of an intravenous barbiturate must be given, as the first effect of suxamethonium is to cause painful muscle contraction before the relaxant action supervenes. Dose 30 to 60 mg repeated as required, or by drip infusion in doses of 50 to 100 mcg per kg body-weight per minute.

S.V.C. Vaginal tablets of acetarsol, 250 mg.

Symmetrel. Amantadine, q.v.

Synalar. Fluocinolone, q.v.

Synkavit. A water-soluble synthetic vitamin K, q.v.

Syntocinon. Synthetic form of oxytocin, q.v.

Syntopressin. Synthetic form of vasopressin, q.v. Used as nasal spray in the treatment of diabetes mellitus.

T

T.E.M. Triethylene melamine or tretamine, q.v.

Tace. Chlorotrianisene, q.v.

Tacitin. Benzoctamine, q.v.

talampicillin. A derivative of ampicillin, q.v., with similar therapeutic applications. High blood-levels are obtained with standard doses of 250 mg three times daily.

talc. Native magnesium silicate. A soft white powder, extensively used as dusting powder. It is also used as lubricant for surgeons' gloves but may cause a talc granuloma if it gains access to the tissues during operations, and the special glove powders prepared from starch are now preferred.

Talpen. Talampicillin, *q.v.*

tamoxifen. A synthetic compound with anti-oestrogenic but not androgenic properties. This selective action is unusual, and the drug is free from the side-effects of androgens used as anti-oestrogens. Of value in the post-menopausal treatment of breast cancer. Dose 10 mg twice daily.

Tanderil. Oxyphenbutazone, *q.v.*

tannic acid. An astringent obtained from oak galls. It is an antidote in acute alkaloid poisoning, and is used for its astringent effects in haemorrhoids as suppositories.

Taractan. Chlorprothixene, *q.v.*

tartar emetic. Antimony and potassium tartrate, *q.v.*

Tavegil. Clemastine, *q.v.*

Tegretol. Carbamazepine, *q.v.*

Telepaque. Iopanoic acid, *q.v.*

Tenuate. Diethylpropion, *q.v.*

terbutaline. A bronchodilator similar in action and uses to salbutamol, *q.v.* Useful in bronchospasm due to allergic or intrinsic asthma.

Teronac. Mazindol, *q.v.*

Terramycin. Oxytetracycline, *q.v.*

Tertroxin. Liothyronine, *q.v.*

testosterone. The androgenic hormone of the testes, which controls the development of the male sex characteristics. Used in male underdevelopment, and gynaecomastia. In the female it is sometimes used to control uterine bleeding, and in large doses is of value in the palliative treatment of certain forms of carcinoma of the breast. Usually given by intramuscular injection as testosterone propionate, but special tablets (100 mg) for implantation in the tissues for a prolonged action are available, as well as tablets for oral use. Dose 10 mg orally, 25 to 100 mg intramuscularly, and 100 to 600 mg by implantation.

Tetmosol. An organic sulphide used by local application in the treatment of scabies.

tetrachlorethylene. An anthelmintic used against hookworms. Dose 3 to 5 ml as a single dose. Owing to possible toxic effects on the liver, the dose should not be repeated in less than ten days.

tetracycline. A wide-range antibiotic very similar both chemically and pharmacologically to chlortetracycline, oxytetracycline, clomocycline and related compounds referred to generically as the tetracyclines. They all have the same type of action against both Gram-positive and Gram-negative organisms, but exhibit certain differences in solubility, absorption and excretion. These differences are reflected in the different doses, as tetracycline is given in doses of 250 mg four times a day, whereas with doxycycline a single daily dose of 250 mg may be adequate. Long treatment with a tetracycline may lead to gastro-intestinal disturbance owing to changes in the normal bacterial population of the intestinal tract.

Tetracyn. Tetracycline, *q.v.*

Thalazole. Phthalylsulphathiazole, *q.v.*

theobromine. An alkaloid similar to caffeine, but with a reduced stimulating action. It has been used in mild hypertension, often in association with phenobarbitone, as in Theominal. Dose 300 to 600 mg.

theophylline. An alkaloid similar to theobromine, but with a more powerful cardiac and diuretic action. Widely used as the more soluble derivative aminophylline, *q.v.*, in asthma and congestive heart failure. Dose 60 to 200 mg.

Thephorin. Phenindamine, *q.v.*

thiabendazole. An anthelmintic effective against a wide range of intestinal parasites. Also useful in creeping eruption. Dose 50 mg/kg daily, up to a maximum of 3 g for one to three days.

thiacetazone. An antitubercular drug of considerable potency, but must be used in conjunction with other drugs to prevent drug resistance. Initial dose 12·5 to 25 mg, increased up to 200 mg daily. Prolonged treatment is necessary, continued after remission of symptoms.

thiambutosine. Used in the treatment of leprosy, as it may have a more rapid initial effect than dapsone, *q.v.* Resistance may occur after prolonged treatment. Dose 500 mg to 2 g daily. Sometimes given by injection in doses of 200 mg to 1 g weekly.

thiamine. Also known as aneurine and vitamin B_1. It is essential for carbohydrate metabolism, but is used clinically mainly in cases of deficiency, as in beri-beri, or when the diet is restricted. Also of value in the neuritis of pregnancy and alcoholism. Prophylactic dose 2 to 5 mg daily; therapeutic dose 25 to 100 mg daily.

Thiazamide. Sulphathiazole, *q.v.*

thiethylperazine. Although related to chlorpromazine, this drug is used only as an anti-emetic, as it has no significant tranquillizing or sedative action. Dose 10 to 30 mg orally, 10 to 20 mg by intra-muscular injection.

thiocarlide. A tuberculostatic drug, used mainly in pul-monary tuberculosis, in combination with other drugs, chiefly in conditions of intolerance to other forms of therapy. Dose 6 to 8 g daily.

thioguanine. An antineoplastic agent similar in action and uses to mercaptopurine. Used in acute and chronic leuk-aemias, in oral doses of 2 mg/kg daily, under close control.

thiomersal. A mercurial anti-septic and fungicide.

thiopentone. A widely used short-acting barbiturate given by intravenous injection for basal narcosis or anaesthesia. Solutions should be freshly prepared. Dose 0·1 to 0·5 g. Great care must be taken to avoid injection outside a vein, as the solution is very alka-line, and may cause necrosis.

thiopropazate. A tranquillizer similar in action to chlorpro-mazine, *q.v.* Useful in agitated and aggressive psychotic patients. Dose 5 to 10 mg.

thioridazine. A tranquillizing drug related to chlorpro-mazine, and used in similar doses for the treatment of various psychiatric condi-tions. Unlike most related drugs, it has no anti-emetic properties. Dose 30 to 600 mg daily.

Thiosporin. A derivative of poly-myxin B, *q.v.*, but less irritat-ing, and more suitable for injection.

thiotepa. A cytotoxic drug similar in action to mustine, *q.v.*, but not irritant. Used in a variety of cancerous condi-tions by various injection routes in doses of 0·2 mg per kg body-weight daily for 3 to 5 days. Larger doses have been injected directly into tumours.

thiothixene. A powerful tran-quillizer for use in schizo-phrenia and paranoid states in adults. Dose 10 mg daily initially, increased to 20 to 30 mg if required.

thymol. A phenolic compound from oil of thyme. Has some antiseptic properties, and is used in mouthwashes, etc.

thymoxamine. A peripheral vasodilator that functions by opposing the vasoconstrictor action of circulatory nor-adrenaline. Useful in a wide range of peripheral ischaemic conditions. Dose 40 mg orally daily, 5 to 30 mg daily by intramuscular or intravenous injection.

thyroid. The dried, defatted gland of the ox, sheep or pig, adjusted with lactose to contain 0·1% iodine, as thyroxine. It is a powerful metabolic stimulant, and is specific in the treatment of myxoedema and cretinism. In the latter condition early diagnosis is essential to obtain full benefit from thyroid therapy and lifelong treatment is necessary. The main hormone, thyroxine, *q.v.*, is now preferred, as absorption is more reliable, and the response more consistent.

thyroxine. The active constituent of thyroid, *q.v.*, but also prepared synthetically. Used in thyroid deficiency states. Initial doses should be small, gradually increased to a suitable maintenance dose. Dose 0·05 to 0·2 mg daily. The response to treatment is slow, and adjustments are made at fortnightly intervals until a metabolic balance and maintenance dose can be assessed.

timolol. A beta-adrenergic blocking agent of the propranolol (*q.v.*) type, used in the control of angina and hypertension. Care is necessary in bradycardia, cardiac insufficiency and bronchial disease. Dose 5 mg thrice daily initially, slowly adjusted to maintenance dose of 15 to 45 mg daily.

tobramycin. An antibiotic of the streptomycin type, active against many Gram-negative organisms. Given by intramuscular injection or intravenous infusion in doses of 3 to 5 mg/kg daily. Care is necessary to avoid the toxic effects of this type of drug.

tocopherol. Also known as vitamin E. Has been given in habitual abortion, in some muscle disorders, and a variety of other conditions, but convincing proof of its value is lacking. Dose 3 to 10 mg.

Tofranil. Imipramine, *q.v.*

Tolanase. Tolazamide, *q.v.*

tolazamide. An oral hypoglycaemic drug related to tolbutamide, *q.v.* Used in late-onset diabetes in doses of 100 to 200 mg daily.

tolazoline hydrochloride. A peripheral vasodilator, exerting its greatest effects on the small vessels of the extremities. It is given in Raynaud's disease and similar conditions; and is used occasionally as drops in keratitis, iritis, etc. Useful by injection to minimize local effects of thiopentone. Tablets of 25 mg; ampoules of 25 mg for intramuscular injection.

tolbutamide. A sulphonyl derivative of urea similar to chlorpropamide, *q.v.* which has the effect of lowering the blood-sugar level and is therefore of value in diabetes. It is effective orally, and appears to act by stimulating the pancreas to produce or release more insulin, as it is effective only when some part of the pancreas is still active. It thus functions as an 'insulin sparer' and not as a substitute. The best results are obtained with middle-aged and mild diabetics normally stabilized on low doses of insulin. Juvenile and severe diabetics are not suitable cases for tolbutamide therapy. Dose, after stabilization, 1 to 3 tablets daily (0·5 to 1·5 g). A return to insulin may be necessary during illness.

Tolnate. Prothipendyl, *q.v.*

Torecan. Thiethylperazine, *q.v.*

tranylcypromine. A monoamine oxidase inhibitor of use in severe depression not responding to other drugs. Dose 20 mg daily initially, increased to 30 mg daily or more according to need.

Trasicor. Oxprenolol, *q.v.*

Trasylol. Aprotinin, *q.v.*

Tremonil. Methixene, *q.v.*

Trenimon. Triaziquone, *q.v.*

Trescatyl. Ethionamide, *q.v.*

tretamine. Has an action similar to mustine, *q.v.*, but is active orally as well as intravenously. Used in Hodgkin's disease, myeloid and lymphatic leukaemia, etc. Dose 2·5 to 5 mg orally, 2 to 3 mg intravenously at intervals, although

large single doses have been given.

Trevintix. Prothionamide, *q.v.*

triamcinolone. One of the steroids of the cortisone type, but differs from the older drug in being more effective in lower dose, and with fewer side-effects. Useful in all conditions requiring cortisone therapy, except adrenal deficiency states, as it has no salt-retaining properties. Dose 4 to 48 mg daily initially, reduced later to a maintenance dose of 8 mg daily or less. Used locally as triamcinolone acetonide in inflamed skin conditions.

triamterene. A powerful diuretic, unrelated to the thiazides, and effective in conditions not responding to those drugs. Triamterene acts mainly on the distal renal tubule, whereas the thiazides act on the proximal tubule. In severe oedematous conditions triamterene and a thiazide diuretic may be given together. Dose 150 to 250 mg daily.

triaziquone. A cytotoxic agent that acts on dividing cells. Used in lymphomas and chronic leukaemias. Dose 0·5 mg orally or intravenously.

trichloracetic acid. Deliquescent crystals, used as a powerful caustic for warts.

trichlorethylene. A liquid similar

to chloroform and used as an inhalation anaesthetic. It is usually given in association with other anaesthetics. It should not be used in closed-circuit anaesthetic apparatus owing to the formation of toxic breakdown products. The drug also has some analgesic properties and small doses inhaled from crushable glass ampoules are valuable in trigeminal neuralgia.

Tricloryl. A derivative of chloral with the sedative properties of the parent drug, but is less irritant to the gastric mucosa. It can therefore be presented as tablets. Dose 0·5 to 1 g.

Tridione. Troxidone, q.v.

trifluoperazine. A tranquillizing drug of the chlorpromazine type, used in a range of mental conditions including psychosis, schizophrenia, hallucinations, and in lower doses for emotional states, nausea, etc. Dose 1 to 25 mg according to need.

Trilene. Trichlorethylene, q.v.

trimeprazine. A phenothiazine derivative with greater anti-allergic and anti-emetic potency than promethazine or chlorpromazine. Valuable in pruritus and many other itching conditions, in pre-medication, in some psychiatric conditions, and as a sedative for children. Dose 10 to 40 mg daily.

trimetaphan. A ganglionic blocking agent with a very brief action. It is used to produce a controllable reduction in blood-pressure during neuro- and vascular surgery when a relatively bloodless field is necessary. It is given by slow intravenous infusion, the dose being governed by the response, which varies very considerably. Frequent determination of blood-pressure during use is essential.

trimipramine. An antidepressant drug similar to imipramine, q.v. Useful when the response to related drugs is inadequate. Dose 25 to 50 mg, increased as required according to need and response.

trimethoprim. An antimalarial drug similar to pyrimethamine, q.v. It also has some antibacterial action, and when given in association with a sulphonamide, the effects are increased, and the risk of bacterial resistance is reduced. That synergistic action is the basis of mixed products such as Septrin and Bactrim.

triperidol. A tranquillizer with properties basically similar to those of chlorpromazine. Useful in chronic schizophrenia. Dose 1·5 to 2·5 mg, daily.

Tromexan. Ethyl biscoumacetate, q.v.

Trophysan. A solution of essential amino-acids, minerals and vitamins for parenteral nutrition when oral feeding is impossible.

troxidone. An anticonvulsant used in petit mal epilepsy. It may cause some toxic effects, including skin rashes, agranulocytosis and photophobia. Initial doses should be small, and increased slowly according to need and response. Dose 0·3 to 2 g daily.

trypsin. A proteolytic enzyme of the pancreas. Highly purified fractions are used by local application for their proteolytic effects, or given by injection in thrombosis and inflammatory conditions. Chymotrypsin is used in ophthalmology.

Tryptizol. Amitriptyline, *q.v.*

tryptophan. An amino-acid present in the diet, that is the precursor of serotonin, *q.v.* A deficiency of serotonin in the brain is associated with some forms of depression, and the administration of tryptophan increases the brain level of serotonin. The response is slow, and some months of treatment is necessary before any relief of depression can be assessed. Dose 1 g three times a day initially, doubled later if required.

Tubarine. Solution of tubocurarine, *q.v.*, containing 10 mg per ml in ampoules of 1·5 ml.

tuberculin. Concentrated filtrate of cultures of *Mycobacterium tuberculosis*. Used in the diagnosis of tuberculosis as Mantoux test.

tubocurarine. The muscle-relaxing constituent of curare. Used in conjunction with general anaesthetics to increase relaxation during surgery; in the treatment of tetanus, and in the convulsive or shock treatment of mental disorders. Dose 10 to 15 mg, intravenously, followed by additional doses if required of 2 to 4 mg at intervals of 25 minutes to a total of 45 mg.

tyrothricin. A mixture of antibiotics derived from cultures of *Bacillus brevis*. Contains gramicidin, *q.v.* It is too toxic for systemic use and is used mainly as lozenges for mouth infections, or as a cream or lotion for burns and skin infections.

U

Ubretid. Distigmine, *q.v.*

Ultrapen. Propicillin, *q.v.*

undecenoic acid. Has useful antimycotic properties. It is used mainly as powder or ointment (5%), often with zinc undecylenate in the treatment of athlete's foot and associated conditions.

Uracil Mustard. Uramustine, *q.v.*

uramustine. A derivative of mustine, *q.v.*, with similar properties. Used in doses of 1 to 2 mg daily for controlled periods in chronic lymphatic leukaemia and lymphoma.

urea. Given intravenously as a 30% solution to reduce cerebral oedema following injury. Has been given orally as a diuretic in doses of 5 to 15 g. A single dose of 15 g is sometimes given to test renal function. Applied locally as a 10% solution, it promotes granulation and reduces odour from foul ulcers.

Urispas. Flavoxate, *q.v.*

Urolucosil. Sulphamethizole, *q.v.*

V

vaccines. Bacterial vaccines are suspensions or extracts of dead bacteria. They may be given by subcutaneous or intramuscular injection, and are used mainly for prophylaxis against a particular infection. The therapeutic use of vaccines, as distinct from prophylaxis, is generally of little value. The most commonly used vaccines include antityphoid-para-typhoid vaccine (T.A.B.), cholera vaccine, staphylococcus vaccine and whooping-cough vaccine. Smallpox vaccine and yellow fever vaccine are prepared from the corresponding viruses. Autogenous vaccines are specially prepared from bacteria cultured from the patient to be treated.

Valium. Diazepam, *q.v.*

Vallergan. Trimeprazine, *q.v.*

Vancocin. Vancomycin, *q.v.*

vancomycin. An antibiotic used in overwhelming staphylococcal infections resistant to other antibiotics. Of no value in infections due to Gram-negative organisms. Dose 2 g daily by slow intravenous injection.

Vandid. Ethamivan, *q.v.*

Vanquin. Viprynium, *q.v.*

Varidase. Preparation of streptokinase, *q.v.* and streptodornase.

vasopressin. A preparation of the blood-pressure-raising and antidiuretic factors of the pituitary gland. Used in paralytic ileus, and diabetes insipidus. Dose 0·5 to 0·75 ml by subcutaneous or intramuscular injection. Pitressin tannate is a long-acting form given by intramuscular injection only.

Vasoxine. Methoxamine, *q.v.*

Vatensol. Guanoclor, *q.v.*

Veganin. Tablets of aspirin, paracetamol and codeine.

Velbe. Vinblastine, *q.v.*

Velosef. Cephradine, *q.v.*

Ventolin. Salbutamol, *q.v.*

Veriloid. Preparations of alkaloids of green hellebore. Occasionally used in hypertension and the toxaemia of pregnancy. Dose 2 mg four times a day, increased up to 12 mg daily.

Vibramycin. Doxycycline. *q.v.*

viloxazine. An antidepressant without sedative effects. Useful in mixed anxiety-repressive states, and in depression in epileptics. May increase the action of phenytoin and antihypertensive agents. Dose 50 to 100 mg thrice daily.

vinblastine. An alkaloid of periwinkle that has cytotoxic properties. Used chiefly in Hodgkin's disease and lung cancer. Dose 0·1 mg per kg body-weight weekly by intravenous injection, increasing by 0·05 mg weekly until adequate response.

vincristine. An alkaloid of periwinkle, used in the treatment of leukaemia in children. Dose 30 to 50 mcg per kg body-weight weekly by intravenous injection.

Vinesthene. Vinyl ether, *q.v.*

vinyl ether. A colourless inflammable liquid, used as an inhalation anaesthetic for minor operations of short duration, and as an induction anaesthetic.

viomycin. An antibiotic derived from cultures of *Streptomyces* spp. Inhibits growth of *M.*

tuberculosis, but owing to toxic effects is used only in cases of resistance to other anti-tuberculous drugs. Dose 1 g twice a day by intramuscular injection together with isoniazid or aminosalicylic acid.

viprynium. An anthelmintic chiefly of value against threadworms. Average adult dose 50 mg. A second dose may be given after 2 to 3 weeks.

vitamin A. One of the vitamins obtained from fish-liver oils. A deficiency in the diet causes night-blindness, skin changes and a decreased resistance to infection. Dose 2,500 to 25,000 units daily.

vitamin B. A name applied to a group of water-soluble vitamins obtained from yeast or rice polishings. The constituents include thiamine, riboflavine, nicotinic acid, pyridoxine, and small amounts of other factors.

vitamin B_{12}. Cyanocobalamin, *q.v.*

vitamin C. Ascorbic acid, *q.v.*

vitamin D. Calciferol, *q.v.*

vitamin E. The vitamin present in wheat-germ oil, now largely replaced by the synthetic form tocopherol, *q.v.*

vitamin K. The vitamin concerned with the formation of prothrombin, and so with blood coagulation. Given as menaphthone, acetomenaphthone or Synkavit in the treatment of haemorrhage due to obstructive jaundice. Vitamin K preparations are of no value in haemorrhage when the prothrombin level of the blood is adequate. Vitamin K_1, or phytomenadione, has a similar but more rapid and sustained action, and is used mainly in the treatment of excessive response to oral anticoagulants. Dose 5 to 20 mg, orally, or by intramuscular or intravenous injection.

Vivalan. Viloxazine, *q.v.*

W

warfarin. A synthetic anticoagulant similar to phenindione, *q.v.*, but with reduced side-effects. It is effective in lower doses, and tablets of 1, 3, 5 and 10 mg are available. Dose is based on the prothrombin level, and is determined on individual requirements.

Welldorm. A derivative of chloral hydrate and phenazone. The product has less gastric irritant effects than chloral, and can be given as tablets, each of which is equivalent to 0·6 g of chloral hydrate.

Whitfield's ointment. Benzoic acid 6%, salicylic acid 3%. Has keratolytic and fungicidal properties, and is used mainly for ringworm.

wintergreen oil. Methyl salicylate, *q.v.*

wool alcohols. A water-in-oil emulsifying agent obtained from wool-fat. It is used in many water-containing ointments, such as ointment of wool alcohols and hydrous ointment.

X

Xylocaine. Lignocaine, *q.v.*

Y

yeast. The fungus used in the fermentation of sugars to produce alcohol. Dried yeast has been used as dietary supplement for its vitamin B content.

Yomesan. Niclosamide, *q.v.*

Z

Zarontin. Ethosuximide, *q.v.*

Zinamide. Pyrazinamide, *q.v.*

zinc oxide. Soft white powder widely used in dusting powders, ointments, pastes, etc., for its mild astringent and antiseptic properties. Constituent of Lassar's paste, Unna's paste, calamine lotion and similar preparations.

zinc peroxide. Insoluble white powder with an antiseptic action similar to hydrogen peroxide but slower and more prolonged. Used as lotion (40%), mouthwash (25%), ointment (20%).

zinc stearate. A white insoluble powder used as a mild astringent in dusting powders for eczema and associated conditions.

zinc sulphate. Used as an astringent and stimulating lotion for indolent ulcers; and in conjunctivitis. Small doses (220 mg) with meals are stated to promote healing of wounds.

zinc undecenoate. White insoluble powder. Constituent of dusting powders and ointments for mycotic conditions.

Zyloric. Allopurinol, *q.v.*

Approved and Proprietary Names of Drugs

APPROVED AND PROPRIETARY NAMES OF DRUGS

New drugs are usually introduced under a brand or proprietary name, but in many cases 'Approved' or non-proprietary names are also in use. The following lists give both the Approved Name and Proprietary Name of a number of available drugs. It does not include mixed products.

Approved Name	Proprietary Name	Main Action, Type of Drug or Use
acebutolol	Sectral	adrenergic blockade
acepifylline	Etophylate	spasmolytic
acetazolamide	Diamox	glaucoma
acetohexamide	Dimelor	oral hypoglycaemic
acetylcysteine	Airbron	mucolytic
alclofenac	Prinalgin	analgesic
alcuronium	Alloferin	muscle-relaxant
aldosterone	Aldocorten	corticosteroid
allopurinol	Zyloric	uricosuric
allyloestrenol	Gestanin	progestogen
aloxiprin	Palaprin	antirheumatic
amantadine	Symmetrel	parkinsonism
ambenonium	Myletase	myasthenia gravis
amiloride	Midamor	diuretic
aminocaproic acid	Epsikapron	haemostatic
amiphenazole	Daptazole	respiratory stimulant
amitriptyline	Laroxyl, Saroten, Tryptizol	antidepressant
amodiaquine	Camoquin	antimalarial
amoxycillin	Amoxil	antibiotic

amphotericin B	Fungizone; Fungilin	antifungal antibiotic
ampicillin	Penbritin; Amfipen, Pentrexyl	antibiotic
ancrod	Arvin	anticoagulant
antazoline	Antistin	antihistamine
aprotinin	Trasylol	enzyme inhibitor
azathioprine	Imuran	antimetabolite; immunosuppressive
baclofen	Lioresal	muscle-relaxant
bamethan	Vasculit	vasodilator
beclamide	Nydrane	anticonvulsant
beclomethasone	Becotide; Propaderm	corticosteroid
bemegride	Megimide	respiratory stimulant
benapryzine	Brizin	parkinsonism
bendrofluazide	Aprinox; Centyl; NeoNaclex	diuretic
benorylate	Benoral	analgesic
benperidol	Anquil	tranquillizer
benzalkonium chloride	Roccal	antiseptic
benzathine penicillin	Penidural	antibiotic
benzhexol	Artane; Pipanol	parkinsonism
benzilonium bromide	Portyn	peptic ulcer
benzoctamine	Tacitin	tranquillizer
benztropine	Cogentin	parkinsonism
bephenium hydroxynaphthoate	Alcopar	anthelmintic
betahistine	Serc	Ménière's disease
betamethasone	Betnelan; Betnovate	corticosteroid
bethanidine	Esbatal	antihypertensive
biperidon	Akineton	parkinsonism

Approved Name	Proprietary Name	Main Action, Type of Drug or Use
bisacodyl	Dulcolax	laxative
bretylium tosylate	Darenthin	antihypertensive
bromhexine	Bisolvon	mucolytic
bromocriptine	Parlodel	anti-lactation, acromegaly
brompheniramine	Dimotane	antihistamine
buclizine	Vibazine	antiemetic
buclosamide	Jadit	antimycotic
bumetanide	Burinex	diuretic
bupivacaine	Marcain	anaesthetic
busulphan	Myleran	antineoplastic
calcitonin	Calcicare	hormone
candicidin	Candeptin	antimycotic
capreomycin	Capastat	antibiotic
carbamazepine	Tegretol	anticonvulsant; analgesic
carbenicillin	Pyopen	antibiotic
carbenoxolone	Biogastrone	peptic ulcer
carbimazole	Neo-Mercazole	thyrotoxicosis
cephalexin	Ceporex; Keflex	antibiotic
cephaloridine	Ceporin	antibiotic
cephalothin	Keflin	antibiotic
cephradine	Eskacef; Velosef	antibiotic
chlorambucil	Leukeran	antineoplastic
chloramphenicol	Chloromycetin	antibiotic
chlordiazepoxide	Librium; Tropium	tranquillizer
chlorhexidine	Hibitane	antiseptic

116

chlormethiazole	Heminevrin	hypnotic
chlormezanone	Trancopal	tranquillizer
chloroquine	Nivaquine; Avloclor	antimalarial
chlorothiazide	Saluric	diuretic
chlorotrianisene	Tace	oestrogen
chlorphenesin	Mycil	antimycotic
chlorpheniramine	Piriton	antihistamine
chlorphenoxamine	Clorevan	parkinsonism
chlorproguanil	Lapudrine	antimalarial
chlorpromazine	Largactil	tranquillizer
chlorpropamide	Diabinese	oral hypoglycaemic
chlorprothixene	Taractan	tranquillizer
chlortetracycline	Aureomycin	antibiotic
chlorthalidone	Hygroton	diuretic
cholestyramine	Cuemid; Questran	bile acid sequestrant
choline theophyllinate	Choledyl	bronchodilator
cinchocaine	Nupercaine	anaesthetic
cinnarizine	Stugeron	antiemetic
clemastine	Tavegil	antihistamine
clindamycin	Dalacin C	antibiotic
clobetasone	Molivate	corticosteroid
clofazimine	Lamprene	antileprotic
clofibrate	Atromid-S	hypercholesterolaemia
clomiphene	Clomid	gonadotrophin inhibitor
clomipramine	Anafranil	antidepressant
clomocycline	Megaclor	antibiotic
clonazepam	Rivotril	anticonvulsant

117

Approved Name	Proprietary Name	Main Action, Type of Drug or Use
clonidine	Catapres; Dixarit	antihypertensive, migraine
clopamide	Brinaldix	diuretic
clorazepic acid	Tranxene	sedative
clorexolone	Nefrolan	diuretic
clotrimazole	Canestan	antimycotic
cloxacillin	Orbenin	antibiotic
colaspase	Crasnitin	antineoplastic
colistin	Colomycin	antibiotic
corticotrophin	ACTH	hormone
crotamiton	Eurax	antipruritic
cyanocobalamin	Cobalin; Cytacon; Cytamen	antianaemic
cyclandelate	Cyclospasmol	vasodilator
cyclizine	Marzine; Valoid	antiemetic
cyclobarbitone	Phanodorm	hypnotic
cyclopenthiazide	Navidrex	diuretic
cyclopentolate	Cyclogyl; Mydrilate	mydriatic
cyclophosphamide	Endoxana	antineoplastic
cyproheptadine	Periactin	antihistamine
cyproterone	Androcur	antiandrogen
cytarabine	Cytosar	antineoplastic
danazol	Danol	pituitary suppressant
danthron	Dorbanex	laxative
dantrolene	Dantrium	muscle-relaxant
daunorubicin	Cerubidin	antibiotic
debrisoquine	Declinax	antihypertensive

118

demecarium bromide	Tosmelin	glaucoma
demeclocycline	Ledermycin	antibiotic
dequalinium chloride	Dequadin	antiseptic
deserpidine	Harmonyl	antihypertensive
desferrioxamine	Desferal	iron poisoning
desipramine	Pertofran	antidepressant
dexamethasone	Decadron; DexaCortisyl; Oradexon	corticosteroid
dexamphetamine	Dexedrine	appetite depressant
dextran	Dextraven; Lomodex; Rheomacrodex	plasma substitute
dextriferron	Astrafer	antianaemic
dextromoramide	Palfium	analgesic
dextropropoxyphene	Doloxene	analgesic
dextrothyroxine	Choloxin	hypercholesterolaemia
diamthazole	Asterol	antimycotic
diazepam	Valium	tranquillizer
diazoxide	Eudemine	antihypertensive
dichloralphenazone	Welldorm	hypnotic
dichlorophen	Anthiphen	anthelmintic
dichlorphenamide	Daranide	glaucoma
dicyclomine	Merbentyl	antispasmodic
diethylcarbamazine	Banocide	filaricide
diethylpropion	Tenuate	appetite depressant
dihydrocodeine	D.F. 118	analgesic
dihydrotachysterol	A.T. 10	hypocalcaemia
di-iodohydroxyquinoline	Diodoquin; Floraquin	amoebiasis

Approved Name	Proprietary Name	Main Action, Type of Drug or Use
diloxanide	Furamide	amoebiasis
dimenhydrinate	Dramamine	antihistamine
dimethisoquin	Quotane	antipruritic
dimethisterone	Secrosteron	progestogen
dinoprost	Prostin F₂	uterine stimulant
dinoprostone	Prostin E₂	uterine stimulant
diphenhydramine	Benadryl	antihistamine
diphenylpyraline	Histryl	antihistamine
dipipanone	Pipadone	analgesic
diprophylline	Neutraphylline; Silbephylline	bronchodilator
dipyridamole	Persantin	vasodilator
disopyramide	Rythmodan	anti-arrhythmic
distigmine	Ubretid	anticholinesterase
disulfiram	Antabuse	alcoholism
domiphen bromide	Bradosol	antiseptic
dothiepin	Prothiaden	antidepressant
doxepin	Sinequan	antidepressant
doxorubicin	Adriamycin	antibiotic
doxycycline	Vibramycin	antibiotic
droperidol	Droleptan	neuroleptic
drostanolone	Masteril	antineoplastic
dydrogesterone	Duphaston	progestogen
ecothiopate	Phospholine	glaucoma
edrophonium chloride	Tensilon	anticholinesterase
emepronium	Cetiprin	anticholinergic

120

erythromycin	Erythrocin; Ilotycin; Erycen	antibiotic
ethacrynic acid	Edecrin	diuretic
ethambutol	Myambutol	tuberculosis
ethamivan	Vandid	respiratory stimulant
ethamsylate	Dicynene	haemostatic
ethchlorvynol	Arrynol; Serenesil	hypnotic
ethebenecid	Urelim	uricosuric
ethionamide	Trescatyl	tuberculosis
ethoglucid	Epodyl	antineoplastic
ethopropazine	Lysivane	parkinsonism
ethosuximide	Emeside; Zarontin	anticonvulsant
ethotoin	Peganone	anticonvulsant
ethyl biscoumacetate	Tromexan	anticoagulant
ethyloestrenol	Orabolin	anabolic steroid
fenfluramine	Ponderax	appetite depressant
fentanyl	Sublimaze	analgesic
flavoxate	Urispas	antispasmodic
flucloxacillin	Floxapen	antibiotic
fludrocortisone	Florinef; Fludrocortone	corticosteroid
flufenamic acid	Arlef	antirheumatic
flumethasone	Locorten	corticosteroid
fluocinolone	Synalar	corticosteroid
fluocinonide	Metosyn	corticosteroid
fluocortolone	Ultralanum	corticosteroid
fluphenazine	Moditen	tranquillizer
flurazepam	Dalamane	hypnotic
fluspirilene	Redeptin	tranquillizer

Approved Name	Proprietary Name	Main Action, Type of Drug or Use
fosfestrol	Honvan	antineoplastic
framycetin	Framygen; Soframycin	antibiotic
frusemide	Lasix	diuretic
furazolidone	Furoxone	intestinal antiseptic
fusidic acid	Fucidin	antibiotic
gallamine	Flaxedil	muscle-relaxant
gefarnate	Gefarnil	peptic ulcer
gentamicin	Cidomycin; Genticin	antibiotic
glibenclamide	Daonil; Euglucon	oral hypoglycaemic
glibornuride	Glutril	oral hypoglycaemic
glipizide	Glibenese, Minodiab	oral hypoglycaemic
glutethimide	Doriden	hypnotic
glymidine	Gondafon	oral hypoglycaemic
griseofulvin	Fulcin; Grisovin	antifungal antibiotic
guanethidine	Ismelin	antihypertensive
guanoclor	Vatensol	antihypertensive
guanoxan	Envacar	antihypertensive
haloperidol	Serenace	tranquillizer
halothane	Fluothane	anaesthetic
heptabarbitone	Medomin	hypnotic
hyaluronidase	Hyalase	enzyme
hydrallazine	Apresoline	antihypertensive
hydrargaphen	Penotrane	antiseptic
hydrochlorothiazide	Direma; Esidrex; Hydrosaluric	diuretic
hydrocortisone	Cortril; Ef-Cortelan;	corticosteroid

122

hydrocortisone	Hydro-cortistab; Hydro-Cortisyl; Hydrocortone	corticosteroid
hydroflumethiazide	Hydrenox	diuretic
hydromorphone	Dilaudid	analgesic
hydroxocobalamin	Neo-Cytamen	antianaemic
hydroxychloroquine	Plaquenil	antimalarial
hydroxyprogesterone	Primolut-Depot	progestogen
hydroxyurea	Hydrea	antineoplastic
hydroxyzine	Atarax	tranquilizer
hyoscine methobromide	Pamine	peptic ulcer
ibuprofen	Brufen	antirheumatic
idoxuridine	Kerecid; Dendrid	antiviral
imipramine	Tofranil	antidepressant
indomethacin	Indocid; Imbrilon	antirheumatic
inositol nicotinate	Hexopal	vasodilator
iodipamide	Biligrafin	contrast agent
iopanoic acid	Telepaque	contrast agent
iophendylate	Myodil	contrast agent
iprindole	Prondol	antidepressant
iproniazid	Marsilid	antidepressant
isocarboxazid	Marplan	antidepressant
isoetharine	Numotac	bronchodilator
isophane insulin	NPH Insulin	hypoglycaemic
isoprenaline	Aleudrin; Neo-Epinine; Saventrine; Suscardia	bronchodilator
isopropamide iodide	Tyrimide	gastric sedative
isoxsuprine	Duvadilan	vasodilator

Approved Name	Proprietary Name	Main Action, Type of Drug or Use
kanamycin	Kannasyn; Kantrex	antibiotic
ketamine	Ketalar	anaesthetic
ketoprofen	Orudis	antirheumatic
lactulose	Duphalac	laxative
levallorphan	Lorfan	narcotic antagonist
levodopa	Brocadopa; Larodopa	parkinsonism
levorphanol	Dromoran	analgesic
lignocaine	Lidothesin; Xylocaine; Xylocard; Xylotox	anaesthetic
lincomycin	Lincocin, Mycivin	antibiotic
liothyronine	Tertroxin	thyroid hormone
loperamide	Imodium	antidiarrhoeal
lorazepam	Ativan	antidepressant
mannomustine	Degranol	antineoplastic
mazindol	Teronac	appetite depressant
mebeverine	Colofac	antispasmodic
mebhydrolin	Fabahistin	antihistamine
mecamylamine	Inversine	antihypertensive
meclofenoxate	Lucidril	cerebral stimulant
medazepam	Nobrium	tranquilizer
mefenamic acid	Ponstan	antirheumatic
mefruside	Baycaron	diuretic
melphalan	Alkeran	antineoplastic
mepenzolate	Cantil	intestinal sedative
mephenesin	Myanesin	muscle-relaxant

mepivacaine	Carbocaine	anaesthetic
meprobamate	Equanil; Mepavlon; Miltown	tranquillizer
mepyramine	Anthisan	antihistamine
mercaptopurine	Puri-Nethol	antineoplastic
metaraminol	Aramine	hypertensive
metformin	Glucophage	oral hypoglycaemic
methacycline	Rondomycin	antibiotic
methadone	Physeptone	analgesic
methallenoestril	Vallestril	oestrogen
methandienone	Dianabol	anabolic steroid
methdilazine	Dilosyn	antihistamine
methenolone	Primobolan	anabolic steroid
methicillin	Celbenin	antibiotic
methisazone	Marboran	antiviral
methixene	Tremonil	parkinsonism
methocarbamol	Robaxin	muscle-relaxant
methohexitone	Brietal	anaesthetic
methoin	Mesontoin	anticonvulsant
methoserpidine	Decaserpyl	antihypertensive
methotrimeprazine	Veractil	tranquillizer
methoxamine	Vasoxine	vasoconstrictor
methoxyflurane	Penthrane	anaesthetic
methoxyphenamine	Orthoxine	bronchodilator
methsuximide	Celontin	anticonvulsant
methyclothiazide	Enduron	diuretic
methylphenidate	Ritalin	stimulant
methyldopa	Aldomet	antihypertensive

Approved Name	Proprietary Name	Main Action, Type of Drug or Use
methylergometrine	Methergin	uterine stimulant
methylpentynol	Oblivon	tranquillizer
methylprednisolone	Medrone	corticosteroid
methyprylone	Noludar	hypnotic
methysergide	Deseril	vasoconstrictor
metoclopramide	Maxolon	antiemetic
metoprolol	Betaloc; Lopresor	adrenergic blockade
metronidazole	Flagyl	trichomoniasis
metyrapone	Metopirone	enzyme inhibitor
mexenone	Uvistat	sunscreen
minocycline	Minocin	antibiotic
naftidrofuryl	Praxilene	vasodilator
nalidixic acid	Negram	urinary antiseptic
nalorphine	Lethidrone	narcotic antagonist
naloxone	Narcan	narcotic antagonist
nandrolone	Deca-Durabolin; Durabolin	anabolic steroid
naphazoline	Privine	decongestant
naproxen	Naprosyn	antirheumatic
natamycin	Pimafucin	antibiotic
nealbarbitone	Censedal	hypnotic
neostigmine	Prostigmin	myasthenia gravis
nialamide	Niamid	antidepressant
niclosamide	Yomesan	anthelmintic
nicotinyl alcohol	Ronicol	vasodilator
nicoumalone	Sinthrome	anticoagulant

126

nifuratel	Magmilor	trichomoniasis
nikethamide	Coramine	respiratory stimulant
niridazole	Ambilhar	schistosomiasis
nitrazepam	Mogadon	hypnotic
nitrofurantoin	Furadantin	urinary antiseptic
nitrofurazone	Furacin	antiseptic
noradrenaline	Levophed	hypertensive
norethandrolone	Nilevar	anabolic steroid
norethisterone	Primulut N	progestogen
nortriptyline	Allegron; Aventyl	antidepressant
novobiocin	Albamycin	antibiotic
noxythiolin	Noxyflex	antiseptic
nystatin	Nystan	antifungal antibiotic
opipramol	Insidon	antidepressant
orciprenaline	Alupent	bronchodilator
orphenadrine	Disipal	parkinsonism
oxazepam	Serenid	tranquillizer
oxolinic acid	Proxodol	urinary antiseptic
oxprenolol	Trasicor	adrenergic blockade
oxycodone	Proladone	analgesic
oxymetholone	Anapolon	anabolic steroid
oxpentifylline	Trental	vasodilator
oxypertine	Integrin	tranquillizer
oxyphenbutazone	Tanderil	antirheumatic
oxyphencyclimine	Daricon	antispasmodic
oxyphenonium	Antrenyl	antispasmodic
oxytetracycline	Berkmycen; Clinimycin;	antibiotic

127

Approved Name	Proprietary Name	Main Action, Type of Drug or Use
oxytetracycline	Imperacin; Stecsolin; Terramycin	antibiotic
pancuronium	Pavulon	muscle-relaxant
paracetamol	Calpol; Febrilix; Panadol	analgesic
paramethadione	Paradione	anticonvulsant
paramethasone	Metilar; Haldrate	corticosteroid
pargyline	Eutonyl	antihypertensive
paromomycin	Humatin	antibiotic
pemoline	Kethamed; Cylert	cerebral stimulant
pempidine	Perolysen	antihypertensive
penicillamine	Distamine; Cuprimine	chelating agent
pentaerythritol tetranitrate	Mycardol; Peritrate	coronary dilator
pentagastrin	Peptavlon	gastric stimulant
pentazocine	Fortral	analgesic
penthienate	Monodral	antispasmodic
pentolinium tartrate	Ansolysen	antihypertensive
pericyazine	Neulactil	tranquillizer
perphenazine	Fentazin	tranquillizer
phenazocine	Narphen	analgesic
phenazopyridine	Pyridium	urinary analgesic
phenelzine	Nardil	antidepressant
phenethicillin	Broxil	antibiotic
pheneturide	Benuride	anticonvulsant
phenformin	Dibotin	oral hypoglycaemic
phenglutarimide	Aturbane	parkinsonism

phenindamine	Thephorin	antihistamine
phenindione	Dindevan	anticoagulant
phenmetrazine	Preludin	appetite suppressant
phenobutiodil	Biliodyl	contrast agent
phenoperidine	Operidine	analgesic
phenoxybenzamine	Dibenyline	adrenaline antagonist
phenoxymethylpenicillin	CVK; Crystapen V; Distaquaine V-K; V-Cil-K	antibiotic
phensuximide	Milontin	anticonvulsant
phentolamine	Rogitine	adrenaline antagonist
phenylbutazone	Butazolidin	antirheumatic
phenylephrine	Neophryn	decongestant
pholcodine	Ethnine	cough suppressant
phytomenadione	Konakion	hypoprothrombinaemia
pimozide	Orap	tranquillizer
pindolol	Visken	coronary dilator
pipenzolate	Piptal	antispasmodic
piperazine	Antepar	anthelmintic
piritamide	Dipidolor	analgesic
poldine	Nacton	antispasmodic
polidexide	Secholex	hypercholesterolaemia
polymyxin B	Aerosporin	antibiotic
polynoxylin	Anaflex	antiseptic
polythiazide	Nephril	diuretic
practolol	Eraldin	adrenergic blockade
prazosin	Hypovase; Sinetens	antihypertensive

129

Approved Name	Proprietary Name	Main Action, Type of Drug or Use
prednisolone	Codelcortone; Delta-Cortef; Deltacortril; Deltastab; Di-Adreson-F; PreCortisyl; Prednesol	corticosteroid
prednisone	DeCortisyl; Deltacortone; Di-Adreson	corticosteroid
prenylamine	Synadrin	coronary dilator
prilocaine	Citanest	anaesthetic
primidone	Mysoline	anticonvulsant
probenecid	Benemid	uricosuric
procainamide	Pronestyl	myocardial depressant
procarbazine	Natulan	antineoplastic
prochlorperazine	Stemetil	tranquillizer
procyclidine	Kemadrin	parkinsonism
prolintane	Villescon	stimulant
promazine	Sparine	tranquillizer
promethazine	Phenergan	antihistamine
promethazine theoclate	Avomine	antiemetic
propanidid	Epontol	anaesthetic
propantheline bromide	Pro-Banthine	anticholinergic
propatylnitrate	Gina	coronary dilator
propicillin	Ultrapen	antibiotic
propranolol	Inderal	adrenergic blockade
propylhexedrine	Benzedrex	decongestant
propyliodone	Dionosil	contrast agent

130

prothionamide	Trevintix	tuberculosis
prothipendyl	Tolnate	tranquilliser
protriptyline	Concordin	antidepressant
proxyphylline	Brontyl	bronchodilator
pyrazinamide	Zinamide	tuberculosis
pyridostigmine	Mestinon	myasthenia gravis
pyrimethamine	Daraprim	antimalarial
quinalbarbitone sodium	Seconal Sodium	hypnotic
quinestradol	Pentovis	oestrogen
quinethazone	Aquamox	diuretic
reserpine	Serpasil	antihypertensive
rifamide	Rifocin-M	antibiotic
rifampicin	Rifadin; Rimactane	antibiotic
rimiterol	Pulmadil	bronchodilator
salbutamol	Ventolin	bronchodilator
sodium acetrizoate	Diaginol	contrast agent
sodium cromoglycate	Intal; Rynacrom	anti-asthmatic
sodium diatrizoate	Hypaque	contrast agent
sodium ipodate	Biloptin	contrast agent
sodium ironedetate	Sytron	antianaemic
sodium valproate	Epilim	anticonvulsant
sorbide nitrate	Vascardin	coronary dilator
sotalol	Beta-Cardone; Sotacor	adrenergic blockade
spectinomycin	Trobicin	antibiotic
spiramycin	Rovamycin	antibiotic
spironolactone	Aldactone-A	diuretic
stanolone	Anabolex	anabolic steroid

131

Approved Name	Proprietary Name	Main Action, Type of Drug or Use
stanozolol	Stromba	anabolic steroid
styramate	Sinaxar	muscle-relaxant
sulfametopyrazine	Kelfizine	sulphonamide
sulphacetamide	Albucid	sulphonamide
sulphadimethoxine	Madribon	sulphonamide
sulphadimidine	Sulphamezathine	sulphonamide
sulphafurazole	Gantrisin	sulphonamide
sulphamethizole	Urolucosil	sulphonamide
sulphamethoxazole	Gantanol	sulphonamide
sulphamethoxydiazine	Durenate	sulphonamide
sulphamethoxpyridazine	Lederkyn; Midicel	sulphonamide
sulphaphenazole	Orisul	sulphonamide
sulphasalazine	Salazopyrin	sulphonamide
sulphinpyrazone	Anturan	uricosuric
sulthiame	Ospolot	anticonvulsant
suxamethonium bromide	Brevidil M	muscle-relaxant
suxamethonium chloride	Anectine	muscle-relaxant
talampicillin	Talpen	antibiotic
tamoxifen	Nolvadex	antineoplastic
terbutaline	Bricanyl	bronchodilator
tetracycline	Achromycin; Steclin; Tetrachel; Tetracyn	antibiotic
thiabendazole	Mintezol	anthelmintic
thiambutosine	Ciba 1906	antileprotic
thiethylperazine	Torecan	antiemetic

132

thiocarlide	Isoxyl	tuberculosis
thioguanine	Lanvis	antineoplastic
thiomersal	Merthiolate	antiseptic
thiopropazate	Dartalan	tranquillizer
thioridazine	Melleril	tranquillizer
thiothixene	Navane	tranquillizer
thymoxamine	Opilon	vasodilator
timolol	Blocadren	adrenergic blockade
tobramycin	Nebcin	antibiotic
tolazamide	Tolanase	oral hypoglycaemic
tolazoline	Priscol	vasodilator
tolbutamide	Rastinon	oral hypoglycaemic
tolnaftate	Tinaderm	antimycotic
tranylcypromine	Parnate	antidepressant
tretinoin	Retin-A	acne
triamcinolone	Adcortyl; Ledercort	corticosteroid
triamterene	Dytac	diuretic
triaziquone	Trenimon	antineoplastic
triclofos	Tricloryl	hypnotic
trifluoperazine	Stelazine	tranquillizer
trifluoperidol	Triperidol	neuroleptic
trimeprazine	Vallergan	antihistamine
trimetaphan	Arfonad	antihypertensive
trimetazidine	Vastarel	vasodilator
trimipramine	Surmontil	antidepressant
triprolidine	Actidil	antihistamine
troxidone	Tridione	anticonvulsant

Approved Name	Proprietary Name	Main Action, Type of Drug or Use
vancomycin	Vancocin	antibiotic
viloxazine	Vivalan	antidepressant
vinblastine	Velbe	antineoplastic
vincristine	Oncovin	antineoplastic
viomycin	Viocin	antibiotic
viprynium embonate	Vanquin	anthelmintic
warfarin	Marevan	anticoagulant
xylometazoline	Otrivine	decongestant
zoxazolamine	Flexin	muscle-relaxant

Proprietary Name	Approved Name	Main Action, Type of Drug or Use
ACTH	corticotrophin	hormone
A.T. 10	dihydrotachysterol	hypocalcaemia
Achromycin	tetracycline	antibiotic
Actidil	triprolidine	antihistamine
Adcortyl	triamcinolone	corticosteroid
Adriamycin	doxorubicin	antibiotic
Adroyd	oxymetholone	anabolic steroid
Aerosporin	polymyxin B	antibiotic
Akineton	biperidon	parkinsonism
Albamycin	novobiocin	antibiotic
Albucid	sulphacetamide	sulphonamide
Alcopar	bephenium	anthelmintic
Aldactone-A	spironolactone	diuretic

Aldocorten	aldosterone	corticosteroid
Aldomet	methyldopa	antihypertensive
Aleudrin	isoprenaline	bronchodilator
Alkeran	melphalan	antineoplastic
Allegron	nortriptyline	antidepressant
Alloferin	alcuronium	muscle-relaxant
Alupent	orciprenaline	bronchodilator
Ambilhar	niridazole	anthelmintic
Amifen	ampicillin	antibiotic
Amoxil	amoxycillin	antibiotic
Anabolex	stanolone	anabolic steroid
Anaflex	polynoxylin	antiseptic
Anafranil	clomipramine	antidepressant
Anapolon	oxymetholone	anabolic steroid
Androcur	cyproterone	pituitary suppressant
Anquil	benperidol	tranquilizer
Ansolysen	pentolinium	antihypertensive
Antabuse	disulfiram	alcoholism
Antepar	piperazine	anthelmintic
Anthiphen	dichlorophen	anthelmintic
Anthisan	mepyramine	antihistamine
Antrenyl	oxyphenonium	antispasmodic
Anturan	sulphinpyrazone	uricosuric
Apresoline	hydrallazine	antihypertensive
Aprinox	bendrofluazide	diuretic
Aquamox	quinethazone	diuretic
Aramine	metaraminol	hypotensive

135

Proprietary Name	Approved Name	Main Action, Type of Drug or Use
Arfonad	trimetaphan	antihypertensive
Arlef	flufenamic acid	antirheumatic
Artane	benzhexol	parkinsonism
Arvin	ancrod	anticoagulant
Arynol	ethchlorvynol	sedative
Asterol	diamthazole	antimycotic
Astrafer	dextriferron	antianaemic
Atarax	hydroxyzine	tranquillizer
Ativan	lorazepam	antidepressant
Atromid-S	clofibrate	hypercholesterolaemia
Aturbane	phenglutarimide	parkinsonism
Aureomycin	chlortetracycline	antibiotic
Aventyl	nortriptyline	antidepressant
Avloclor	chloroquine	antimalarial
Avomine	promethazine theoclate	antiemetic
Banocide	diethylcarbamazine	filaricide
Baycaron	mefruside	diuretic
Becotide	beclomethasone	corticosteroid
Benadryl	diphenhydramine	antihistamine
Benemid	probenecid	uricosuric
Benoral	benorylate	analgesic
Benuride	pheneturide	anticonvulsant
Benzedrex	propylhexedrine	decongestant
Berkmycen	oxytetracycline	antibiotic
Berkomine	imipramine	antidepressant

Beta-Cardone	sotalol	adrenergic blockade
Betaloc	metoprolol	adrenergic blockade
Betnelan	betamethasone	corticosteroid
Biligrafin	iodipamide	contrast agent
Biliodyl	phenobutiodil	contrast agent
Biloptin	sodium ipodate	contrast agent
Biogastrone	carbenoxolone	peptic ulcer
Bisolvon	bromhexine	mucolytic
Blocadren	timolol	adrenergic blockade
Bradosol	domiphen	antiseptic
Brevidil M	suxamethonium bromide	muscle-relaxant
Bricanyl	terbutaline	bronchodilator
Brietal	methohexitone	anaesthetic
Brinaldix	clopamide	diuretic
Brizin	benapryzine	parkinsonism
Brocadopa	levodopa	parkinsonism
Brocillin	propicillin	antibiotic
Brontyl	proxyphylline	bronchodilator
Broxil	phenethicillin	antibiotic
Burinex	bumetanide	diuretic
Butazolidin	phenylbutazone	antirheumatic
Calcicare	calcitonin	hormone
Calpol	paracetamol	analgesic
Camoquin	amodiaquine	antimalarial
Candeptin	candicidin	antibiotic
Canestan	clotrimazole	antimycotic
Cantil	mepenzolate	intestinal sedative

Proprietary Name	Approved Name	Main Action, Type of Drug or Use
Capastat	capreomycin	tuberculosis
Carbocaine	mepivacaine	anaesthetic
Celbenin	methicillin	antibiotic
Celontin	methsuximide	anticonvulsant
Censedal	nealbarbitone	hypnotic
Centyl	bendrofluazide	diuretic
Ceporex	cephalexin	antibiotic
Ceporin	cephaloridine	antibiotic
Cerubidin	daunorubicin	antineoplastic
Cetiprin	emepronium	anticholinergic
Chloromycetin	chloramphenicol	antibiotic
Chlor-Trimeton	chlorpheniramine	antihistamine
Choledyl	choline theophyllinate	bronchodilator
Choloxin	dextrothyroxine	hypercholesterolaemia
Cidomycin	gentamicin	antibiotic
Citanest	prilocaine	anaesthetic
Clinimycin	oxytetracycline	antibiotic
Clinitetrin	tetracycline	antibiotic
Clomid	clomiphene	gonadotrophin inhibitor
Clorevan	chlorphenoxamine	parkinsonism
Codelcortone	prednisolone	corticosteroid
Cogentin	benztropine	parkinsonism
Colofac	mebeverine	antispasmodic
Colomycin	colistin	antibiotic
Concordin	protriptyline	antidepressant

138

Compocillin-VK	phenoxymethylpenicillin	antibiotic
Coramine	nikethamide	respiratory stimulant
Cortef	hydrocortisone	corticosteroid
Cortril	hydrocortisone	corticosteroid
Cortrophin	corticotrophin	hormone
Crasnitin	colaspase	antineoplastic
Crystapen V	phenoxymethylpenicillin	antibiotic
Cuemid	cholestyramine	bile acid sequestrant
Cuprimine	penicillamine	chelating agent
Cyclogyl	cyclopentolate	mydriatic
Cyclospasmol	cyclandelate	vasodilator
Cylert	pemoline	cerebral stimulant
Cytacon	cyanocobalamin	antianaemic
Cytamen	cyanocobalamin	antianaemic
Cytosar	cytarabine	antineoplastic
D.F. 118	dihydrocodeine	analgesic
Dalacin C	clindamycin	antibiotic
Dalmane	flurazepam	hypnotic
Danol	danazol	pituitary depressant
Dantrium	dantrolene	muscle-relaxant
Daonil	glibenclamide	oral hypoglycaemic
Daptazole	amiphenazole	respiratory stimulant
Daranide	dichlorphenamide	glaucoma
Daraprim	pyrimethamine	antimalarial
Darenthin	bretylium tosylate	antihypertensive
Daricon	orphencyclimine	antispasmodic
Dartalan	thiopropazate	tranquillizer

Proprietary Name	Approved Name	Main Action, Type of Drug or Use
Decadron	dexamethasone	corticosteroid
Deca-Durabolin	nandrolone	anabolic steroid
Decaserpyl	methoserpidine	antihypertensive
Declinax	debrisoquine	antihypertensive
DeCortisyl	prednisone	corticosteroid
Degranol	mannomustine	antineoplastic
Delta-Cortef	prednisolone	corticosteroid
Deltacortone	prednisone	corticosteroid
Deltacortril	prednisolone	corticosteroid
Dendrid	idoxuridine	antiviral
Depamine	penicillamine	chelating agent
Dequadin	dequalinium	antiseptic
Deseril	methysergide	vasoconstrictor
Desferal	desferrioxamine	chelating agent
DexaCortisyl	dexamethasone	corticosteroid
Dexedrine	dexamphetamine	appetite depressant
Dextraven	dextran	plasma substitute
Diabinese	chlorpropamide	oral hypoglycaemic
Di-Adreson	prednisone	corticosteroid
Di-Adreson-F	prednisolone	corticosteroid
Diaginol	sodium acetrizoate	contrast agent
Diamox	acetazolamide	glaucoma
Dianabol	methandienone	anabolic steroid
Dibenyline	phenoxybenzamine	adrenaline antagonist
Dibotin	phenformin	oral hypoglycaemic

Dicynene	ethamsylate	haemostatic
Dilaudid	hydromorphone	analgesic
Dilavase	isoxsuprine	vasodilator
Dilosyn	methdilazine	antihistamine
Dimelor	acetohexamide	oral hypoglycaemic
Dimotane	brompheniramine	antihistamine
Dindevan	phenindione	anticoagulant
Diodoquin	di-iodohydroxyquinoline	amoebiasis
Dionosil	propyliodone	contrast agent
Di-paralene	chlorcyclizine	antihistamine
Dipidolor	piritamide	analgesic
Direma	hydrochlorothiazide	diuretic
Disipal	orphenadrine	parkinsonism
Distamine	penicillamine	chelating agent
Distaquaine V-K	phenoxymethylpenicillin	antibiotic
Dixarit	clonidine	antihypertensive, migraine
Doloxene	dextropropoxyphene	analgesic
Dorbanex	danthron	laxative
Doriden	glutethimide	hypnotic
Dramamine	dimenhydrinate	antihistamine
Droleptan	droperidol	analgesic
Dromoran	levorphanol	analgesic
Dulcolax	bisacodyl	laxative
Duogastrone	carbenoxolone	peptic ulcer
Duphalac	lactulose	laxative
Duphaston	dydrogesterone	progestogen
Durabolin	nandrolone	anabolic steroid

Proprietary Name	Approved Name	Main Action, Type of Drug or Use
Durenate	sulphamethoxydiazine	sulphonamide
Duvadilan	isoxsuprine	vasodilator
Dytac	triamterene	diuretic
Edecrin	ethacrynic acid	diuretic
Ef-Cortelan	hydrocortisone	corticosteroid
Emeside	ethosuximide	anticonvulsant
Endografin	iodipamide	contrast agent
Endoxana	cyclophosphamide	antineoplastic
Enduron	methyclothiazide	diuretic
Entacyl	piperazine	anthelmintic
Envacar	guanoxan	antihypertensive
Epodyl	ethoglucid	antineoplastic
Epontol	propanidid	anaesthetic
Epsikapron	aminocaproic acid	haemostatic
Equanil	meprobamate	tranquilizer
Eraldin	practolol	adrenergic blockade
Erycen	erythromycin	antibiotic
Erythrocin	erythromycin	antibiotic
Esbatal	bethanidine	antihypertensive
Esidrex	hydrochlorothiazide	diuretic
Eskacef	cephradine	antibiotic
Ethnine	pholcodine	cough suppressant
Etophylate	acephylline	bronchodilator
Eudemine	diazoxide	antihypertensive
Euglucon	glibenclamide	oral hypoglycaemic

142

Eurax	crotamiton	antipruritic
Eutonyl	pargyline	antihypertensive
Fabahistin	mebhydrolin	antihistamine
Febrilix	paracetamol	analgesic
Fentazin	perphenazine	tranquillizer
Flagyl	metronidazole	trichomoniasis
Flaxedil	gallamine	muscle-relaxant
Flexin	zoxazolamine	muscle-relaxant
Floraquin	di-iodohydroxyquinoline	antiamoebic
Florinef	fludrocortisone	corticosteroid
Floxapen	flucloxacillin	antibiotic
Fludrocortone	fludrocortisone	corticosteroid
Fluothane	halothane	anaesthetic
Fortral	pentazocine	analgesic
Framygen	framycetin	antibiotic
Fucidin	fusidic acid	antibiotic
Fulcin	griseofulvin	antifungal antibiotic
Fungilin	amphotericin-B	antifungal antibiotic
Fungizone	amphotericin-B	antifungal antibiotic
Furacin	nitrofurazone	antiseptic
Furadantin	nitrofurantoin	urinary antiseptic
Furamide	diloxanide	antiamoebic
Furoxone	furazolidone	intestinal antiseptic
Gantanol	sulphamethoxazole	sulphonamide
Gantrisin	sulphafurazole	sulphonamide
Gefarnil	gefarnate	peptic ulcer
Genticin	gentamicin	antibiotic

143

Proprietary Name	Approved Name	Main Action, Type of Drug or Use
Gestanin	allyloestrenol	progestogen
Gina	propatylnitrate	coronary dilator
Glibenese	glipizide	oral hypoglycaemic
Glucophage	metformin	oral hypoglycaemic
Glutril	glibornuride	oral hypoglycaemic
Gondafon	glymidine	oral hypoglycaemic
Grisovin	griseofulvin	antifungal antibiotic
Haldrate	paramethasone	corticosteroid
Harmonyl	deserpidine	antihypertensive
Heminevrin	chlormethiazole	hypnotic
Hexopal	inositol nicotinate	vasodilator
Hibitane	chlorhexidine	antiseptic
Histryl	diphenylpyraline	antihistamine
Honvan	fosfestrol	antineoplastic
Humatin	paromomycin	antibiotic
Hyalase	hyaluronidase	enzyme
Hydrea	hydroxyurea	antineoplastic
Hydrenox	hydroflumethiazide	diuretic
Hydro-Cortisyl	hydrocortisone	corticosteroid
Hydrocortone	hydrocortisone	corticosteroid
Hydrosaluric	hydrochlorothiazide	diuretic
Hygroton	chlorthalidone	diuretic
Hypaque	sodium diatrizoate	contrast agent
Hypovase	prazocin	antihypertensive
Icipen V	phenoxymethylpenicillin	antibiotic

Ilosone	erythromycin estolate	antibiotic
Ilotycin	erythromycin	antibiotic
Imbrilon	indomethacin	antirheumatic
Imodium	loperamide	antidiarrhoeal
Imperacin	oxytetracycline	antibiotic
Imuran	azathioprine	immunosuppressive
Inderal	propranolol	adrenergic blockade
Indocid	indomethacin	antirheumatic
Insidon	opipramol	antidepressant
Insulin Lente	insulin zinc suspension	hypoglycaemic
Insulin Semilente	insulin zinc suspension (Amorphous)	hypoglycaemic
Insulin Ultralente	insulin zinc suspension (Crystalline)	hypoglycaemic
Intal	sodium cromoglycate	anti-asthmatic
Integrin	oxypertine	tranquillizer
Inversine	mecamylamine	antihypertensive
Ismelin	guanethidine	antihypertensive
Isoxyl	thiocarlide	tuberculosis
Isupren	isoprenaline	bronchodilator
Jadit	buclosamide	antimycotic
Kannasyn	kanamycin	antibiotic
Kantrex	kanamycin	antibiotic
Kelfizine	sulfametopyrazine	sulphonamide
Kemadrin	procyclidine	parkinsonism
Kerecid	idoxuridine	antiviral
Kethamed	pemoline	cerebral stimulant

145

Proprietary Name	Approved Name	Main Action, Type of Drug or Use
Konakion	phytomenadione	hypoprothrombinaemia
Lamprene	clofazimine	antileprotic
Lanvis	thioguanine	antineoplastic
Lapudrine	chlorproguanil	antimalarial
Largactil	chlorpromazine	tranquillizer
Larodopa	levodopa	parkinsonism
Laroxyl	amitriptyline	antidepressant
Lasix	frusemide	diuretic
Ledercort	triamcinolone	corticosteroid
Lederkyn	sulphamethoxypyridazine	sulphonamide
Ledermycin	demeclocycline	antibiotic
Lethidrone	nalorphine	narcotic antagonist
Leukeran	chlorambucil	antineoplastic
Levophed	noradrenaline	hypertensive
Levorphan	levorphanol	narcotic antagonist
Librium	chlordiazepoxide	tranquillizer
Lidothesin	lignocaine	anaesthetic
Lincocin	lincomycin	antibiotic
Lioresal	baclofen	muscle-relaxant
Locorten	flumethasone	corticosteroid
Lopresor	metoprolol	adrenergic blockade
Lorfan	levallorphan	narcotic antagonist
Lucidril	meclofenoxate	cerebral stimulant
Lysivane	ethopropazine	parkinsonism
Madribon	sulphadimethoxine	sulphonamide

146

Magmilor	nifuratel	trichomoniasis
Marboran	methisazone	antiviral
Marcain	bupivacaine	anaesthetic
Marevan	warfarin	anticoagulant
Marplan	isocarboxazid	antidepressant
Marsilid	iproniazid	antidepressant
Masteril	drostanolone	antineoplastic
Maxolon	metoclopramide	antiemetic
Medomin	heptabarbitone	hypnotic
Medrone	methylprednisolone	corticosteroid
Megaclor	clomocycline	antibiotic
Megimide	bemegride	respiratory stimulant
Melleril	thioridazine	tranquillizer
Mepavlon	meprobamate	tranquillizer
Merbentyl	dicyclomine	antispasmodic
Merthiolate	thiomersal	antiseptic
Mesontoin	methoin	anticonvulsant
Mestinon	pyridostigmine	myasthenia
Methergin	methylergometrine	uterine stimulant
Metilar	paramethasone	corticosteroid
Metopirone	metyrapone	enzyme inhibitor
Metosyn	fluocinonide	corticosteroid
Midicel	sulphamethoxypyridazine	sulphonamide
Midamor	amiloride	diuretic
Minodiab	glipizide	oral hypoglycaemic
Milontin	phensuximide	anticonvulsant
Miltown	meprobamate	tranquillizer

Proprietary Name	Approved Name	Main Action, Type of Drug or Use
Minocin	minocycline	antibiotic
Moditen	fluphenazine	tranquillizer
Mogadon	nitrazepam	hypnotic
Molivate	clobetasone	cortocosteroid
Monodral	penthienate	antispasmodic
Myanesin	mephenesin	muscle-relaxant
Mycardol	pentaerythritol tetranitrate	coronary dilator
Mycil	chlorphenesin	antimycotic
Mycivin	lincomycin	antibiotic
Mydrilate	cyclopentolate	mydriatic
Myleran	busulphan	antineoplastic
Myodil	iophendylate	contrast agent
Mysoline	primidone	anticonvulsant
Mysteclin	tetracycline	antibiotic
Mytelase	ambenonium	myasthenia gravis
NPH Insulin	isophane insulin	hypoglycaemic
Nacton	poldine	antispasmodic
Naprosyn	naproxen	antirheumatic
Narcan	naloxone	narcotic antagonist
Nardil	phenelzine	antidepressant
Narphen	phenazocine	analgesic
Natulan	procarbazine	antineoplastic
Navane	thiothixene	tranquillizer
Navidrex	cyclopenthiazide	diuretic
Nebcin	tobramycin	antibiotic

148

Nefrolan	clorexolone	diuretic
Negram	nalidixic acid	urinary antiseptic
Neo-Cytamen	hydroxocobalamin	antianaemic
Neo-Epinine	isoprenaline	bronchodilator
Neo-Mercazole	carbimazole	thyrotoxicosis
Neo-Naclex	bendrofluazide	diuretic
Neophryn	phenylephrine	decongestant
Nephril	polythiazide	diuretic
Neulactil	pericyazine	tranquillizer
Neutraphylline	diprophylline	bronchodilator
Niamid	nialamide	antidepressant
Nilevar	norethandrolone	anabolic steroid
Nivaquine	chloroquine	antimalarial
Nivemycin	neomycin	antibiotic
Nobrium	medazepam	tranquilliser
Noludar	methyprylone	hypnotic
Nolvadex	tamoxifen	antineoplastic
Norflex	orphenadrine	muscle-relaxant
Nupercaine	cinchocaine	anaesthetic
Nydrane	beclamide	anticonvulsant
Nystan	nystatin	antifungal antibiotic
Oblivon	methylpentynol	tranquilliser
Ocusol	sulphacetamide	sulphonamide
Oncovin	vincristine	antineoplastic
Operidine	phenoperidine	analgesic
Opilon	thymoxamine	vasodilator
Orabolin	ethylestrenol	anabolic steroid

149

Proprietary Name	Approved Name	Main Action, Type of Drug or Use
Oradexon	dexamethasone	corticosteroid
Orap	pimozide	tranquillizer
Orbenin	cloxacillin	antibiotic
Orisulf	sulphaphenazole	sulphonamide
Orthoxine	methoxyphenamine	bronchodilator
Orudis	ketoprofen	antirheumatic
Ospolot	sulthiame	anticonvulsant
Otrivine	xylometazoline	decongestant
Palfium	dextromoramide	analgesic
Pamine	hyoscine methobromide	antispasmodic
Panadol	paracetamol	analgesic
Paradione	paramethadione	anticonvulsant
Parlodel	bromocriptine	anti-lactation, acromegaly
Parnate	tranylcypromine	antidepressant
Pavulon	pancuronium	muscle-relaxant
Peganone	ethotoin	anticonvulsant
Penbritin	ampicillin	antibiotic
Penicillin V	phenoxymethylpenicillin	antibiotic
Penidural	benzathine penicillin	antibiotic
Penotrane	hydrargaphen	antiseptic
Penthrane	methoxyflurane	anaesthetic
Pentovis	quinestradol	oestrogen
Pentrexyl	ampicillin	antibiotic
Peptavlon	pentagastrin	gastric stimulant
Periactin	cyproheptadine	antihistamine

150

Peritrate	pentaerythritol tetranitrate	coronary dilator
Perolysen	pempidine	antihypertensive
Persantin	dipyridamole	vasodilator
Pertofran	desipramine	antidepressant
Phanodorm	cyclobarbitone	hypnotic
Phenergan	promethazine	antihistamine
Phospholine	ecothiopate	glaucoma
Physeptone	methadone	analgesic
Pimafucin	natamycin	antibiotic
Pipadone	dipipanone	analgesic
Pipanol	benzhexol	parkinsonism
Piptal	pipenzolate	antispasmodic
Piriton	chlorpheniramine	antihistamine
Plaquenil	hydroxychloroquine	antimalarial
Ponderax	fenfluramine	appetite depressant
Ponstan	mefenamic acid	antirheumatic
Portyn	benzilonium bromide	antispasmodic
Praxilene	naftidrofuryl	vasodilator
PreCortisyl	prednisolone	corticosteroid
Prednesol	prednisolone	corticosteroid
Preludin	phenmetrazine	appetite depressant
Primobolan	methenolone	anabolic steroid
Primolut N	norethisterone	progestogen
Primolut	hydroxyprogesterone	progestogen
Prinalgin	alclofenac	antirheumatic
Priscol	tolazoline	vasodilator
Privine	naphazoline	decongestant

Proprietary Name	Approved Name	Main Action, Type of Drug or Use
Pro-Banthine	propantheline	anticholinergic
Prodoxol	oxolinic acid	urinary antiseptic
Proladone	oxycodone	analgesic
Prondol	iprindole	antidepressant
Pronestyl	procainamide	myocardial depressant
Propaderm	beclomethasone	corticosteroid
Prostigmin	neostigmine	myasthenia
Prostin E_2	dinoprost	uterine stimulant
Prostin F_2	dinoprostone	uterine stimulant
Pulmadil	rimeritol	bronchodilator
Puri-Nethol	mercaptopurine	antineoplastic
Pyopen	carbenicillin	antibiotic
Pyridium	phenazopyridine	urinary analgesic
Questran	cholestyramine	bile acid sequestrant
Quotane	dimethisoquin	antipruritic
Rastinon	tolbutamide	oral hypoglycaemic
Redeptin	fluspiriline	tranquillizer
Rifadin	rifampicin	tuberculosis
Rifocin-M	rifamide	tuberculosis
Rimactane	rifampicin	tuberculosis
Ritalin	methyl phenidate	central stimulant
Rivotril	clonazepam	anticonvulsant
Robaxin	methocarbamol	muscle-relaxant
Roccal	benzalkonium	antiseptic
Rogitine	phentolamine	adrenaline antagonist

Rondomycin	methacycline	antibiotic
Ronicol	nicotinyl alcohol	vasodilator
Rovamycin	spiramycin	antibiotic
Rythmodan	disopyramide	anti-arrhythmic
Salazopyrin	sulphasalazine	sulphonamide
Saluric	chlorothiazide	diuretic
Saroten	amitriptyline	antidepressant
Saventrine	isoprenaline	bronchodilator
Scoline	suxamethonium chloride	muscle-relaxant
Secholex	polydexide	hypercholesterolaemia
Seconal	quinalbarbitone	hypnotic
Secrosteron	dimethisterone	progestogen
Sectral	acebutolol	adrenergic blockade
Serc	betahistine	Ménière's disease
Serenace	haloperidol	tranquillizer
Serensil	ethchlorvynol	hypnotic
Serenid	oxazepam	tranquillizer
Serpasil	reserpine	antihypertensive
Silbephylline	diprophylline	bronchodilator
Sinaxar	styramate	muscle-relaxant
Sinetens	prazosin	antihypertensive
Sinthrome	nicoumalone	anticoagulant
Soframycin	framycetin	antibiotic
Sotacor	sotalol	adrenergic blockade
Sparine	promazine	tranquillizer
Steclin	tetracycline	antibiotic
Stecsolin	oxytetracycline	antibiotic

Proprietary Name	Approved Name	Main Action, Type of Drug or Use
Stelazine	trifluoperazine	tranquillizer
Stemetil	prochlorperazine	tranquillizer, antiemetic
Stromba	stanozolol	anabolic steroid
Stugeron	cinnarizine	antiemetic
Sublimase	fentanyl	analgesic
Sulphamezathine	sulphadimidine	sulphonamide
Surmontil	trimipramine	antidepressant
Suscardia	isoprenaline	bronchodilator
Symmetrel	amantadine	parkinsonism
Synadrin	prenylamine	coronary dilator
Synalar	fluocinolone	corticosteroid
Sytron	sodium ironedetate	antianaemic
Tace	chlorotrianisene	oestrogen
Tacitin	benzoctamine	tranquillizer
Talpen	talampicillin	antibiotic
Tanderil	oxyphenbutazone	antirheumatic
Taractan	chlorprothixene	tranquillizer
Tavegil	clemastine	antihistamine
Tegretol	carbamazepine	anticonvulsant, analgesic
Telepaque	iopanoic acid	contrast agent
Tensilon	edrophonium	anticholinesterase
Tenuate	diethylpropion	appetite depressant
Teronac	mazindol	appetite depressant
Terramycin	oxytetracycline	antibiotic
Tertroxin	liothyronine	hormone

Tetracyn	tetracycline	antibiotic
Thephorin	phenindamine	antihistamine
Thytropar	thyrotrophin	hormone
Tigloidine	tigloidine	spasmolytic
Tofranil	imipramine	antidepressant
Tolanase	tolazamide	oral hypoglycaemic
Tolnate	prothipendyl	antiemetic
Torecan	thiethylperazine	antiemetic
Tosmelin	demecarium bromide	glaucoma
Trancopal	chlormezanone	tranquillizer
Tranxene	clorazepic acid	sedative
Trasicor	oxprenolol	adrenergic blockade
Trasylol	aprotinin	enzyme inhibitor
Tremonil	methixene	parkinsonism
Trenimon	triaziquone	antineoplastic
Trental	oxypentifylline	bronchodilator
Trescatyl	ethionamide	tuberculosis
Trevintix	prothionamide	tuberculosis
Tricloryl	triclofos	hypnotic
Tridione	troxidone	anticonvulsant
Triperidol	trifluperidol	tranquillizer
Trobicin	spectinomycin	antibiotic
Tromexan	ethyl biscoumacetate	anticoagulant
Tropium	chlordiazepoxide	tranquillizer
Tryptizol	amitriptyline	antidepressant
Tyrimide	isopropamide	gastric sedative
Ubretid	dystigmine	anticholinesterase

155

Proprietary Name	Approved Name	Main Action, Type of Drug or Use
Ultracortenol	prednisolone	corticosteroid
Ultralanum	fluocortelone	corticosteroid
Ultrapen	propicillin	antibiotic
Urelim	ethebenecid	uricosuric
Urispas	flavoxate	antispasmodic
Urolucosil	sulphamethizole	sulphonamide
Uvistat	mexenone	sun screen
V-Cil-K	phenoxymethylpenicillin	antibiotic
Valium	diazepam	tranquillizer
Vallergan	trimeprazine	antihistamine
Vallestril	methallenoestril	oestrogen
Valoid	cyclizine	antiemetic
Vancocin	vancomycin	antibiotic
Vandid	ethamivan	respiratory stimulant
Vanquin	viprynium embonate	anthelmintic
Vascardin	sorbide nitrate	coronary dilator
Vasculit	bamethan	vasodilator
Vastarel	trimetazidine	vasodilator
Vasylox	methoxamine	decongestant
Vatensol	guanoclor	antihypertensive
Velbe	vinblastine	antineoplastic
Velosef	cephradine	antibiotic
Ventolin	salbutamol	bronchodilator
Veractil	methotrimeprazine	tranquillizer
Vibramycin	doxycycline	antibiotic

Villescon	prolintane	stimulant
Viocin	viomycin	antibiotic
Vionactane	viomycin	antibiotic
Visken	pindolol	coronary dilator
Vitamin B_{12}	cyanocobalamin	antianaemic
Vitamin K_1	phytomenadione	hypoprothrombinaemia
Vivalan	viloxazine	antidepressant
Welldorm	dichloralphenazone	hypnotic
Xylocaine	lignocaine	anaesthetic
Xylocard	lignocaine	anti-arrhythmic
Xylotox	lignocaine	anaesthetic
Yomesan	niclosamide	anthelmintic
Zarontin	ethosuximide	anticonvulsant
Zinamide	pyrazinamide	tuberculosis
Zyloric	allopurinol	uricosuric